BARBORI GARNET

The Gift of Journaling

Writing as a Path to Discovery

First published by Garnet Creek Productions 2024

Copyright © 2024 by Barbori Garnet

All rights reserved. No part of this publication may be reproduced, stored or transmitted in any form or by any means, electronic, mechanical, photocopying, recording, scanning, or otherwise without written permission from the publisher. It is illegal to copy this book, post it to a website, or distribute it by any other means without permission.

Barbori Garnet has no responsibility for the persistence or accuracy of URLs for external or third-party Internet Websites referred to in this publication and does not guarantee that any content on such Websites is, or will remain, accurate or appropriate.

First edition

ISBN: 978-1-7382292-0-8

This book was professionally typeset on Reedsy.
Find out more at reedsy.com

To my mother, Barboria.
Thank you for being there at each stage of this journey.

To Matthew.
Thank you for your support and encouragement.

Vision is not enough; it must be combined with venture. It is not enough to stare up the steps; we must step up the stairs.

- Vaclav Havel

Contents

Foreword iv
Introduction vii

I   Part 1: Create Your Journaling Routine

1. Photo Gallery - Journaling Locations and Tools   3
2. The Benefits of Journaling   9
3. Create a Routine   20
4. Remember to Make Journaling a Relaxing and Special Time   24
5. Obstacles to Journaling (and How to Minimize or Remove Them)   31
6. Being Part of a Community and Finding Support   40
7. Journaling - For Men   43
8. Journaling Through…   51
9. Journaling Do's and Don'ts   57

II   Part 2: Types of Journals

10. Career/Work/Business Journal   61
11. Creativity Journal   75
12. Dream Journal   85
13. Education/Learning Journal   88
14. Family History Journal   94

15	Gardening/Home Journal	97
16	Goals Journal	101
17	Gratitude Journal	106
18	Health Journal	110
19	Interests Journal	117
20	Life Journal	123
21	Money/Finance Journal	129
22	Nature Journal	134
23	Prayer/Faith/Bible Journal	138
24	Travel Journal	142

III	Part 3: Hands-on Workbook - How to Sustain Your Journaling Practice	

25	The Place and Space Where You Journal	149
26	Goals and Reasons for Journaling	153
27	Time to Journal	156
28	Socialization and Support Systems	159
29	Health and Wellness	163

IV	Resources	

30	Books	169
31	Websites	172
32	Dualities	173
33	Days and Holidays to Journal About	175
34	Journal Prompts and Questions	176
35	A to Z of Journaling Prompts	178
36	Journal to Rise (aka Start Your Day)	184
37	Journal to Bed (aka Finish Your Day)	185
38	Sample Journaling Retreat Day	186

39	Article - Journaling for Writers	188
40	Article - Support Your Health with a Health Journal	190
41	Book Club Discussion Guide	193
42	A Little Help from Friends and Readers	194

V   Index

43	Index	197

About the Author — 204
Also by Barbori Garnet — 205

Foreword

Foreword by Lynda Monk

The Gift of Journaling: Writing as a Path to Discovery by Barbori Garnet is a gift to those who are avid journal writers and those interested in learning how to create a meaningful journaling practice in their lives.

Like the author, I have been a journal writer since I was a young girl. I was barely past the age of learning to write when I started my first diary. I can still remember my small pink diary with the lock and key. I would hide it away safely in my bedroom, never wanting anyone to find it - or more specifically, read it. I learned at a young age the value of putting my thoughts and feelings down on paper. It has always felt restoring and refreshing to write in the personal, open, honest, and self-expressive way that journaling allows for. As Barbori writes, "Journaling is more than just putting pen to paper to fill the page or the pages of a notebook. Journaling is about a deeper connection to and knowledge of yourself."

People often want to journal, but aren't sure what to write about or how to overcome obstacles along the way. In this book, Barbori addresses some of the common obstacles and offers ways to deal with them that are easy to do. This can help any journal writer to write consistently and with a sense of purpose in mind.

The Gift of Journaling explores not only what journaling is and the many benefits of putting pen to paper, but also offers practical descriptions of various types of journals and specific journaling methods. Each chapter contains inspirational and thoughtful quotes, thought-provoking ideas about journaling, and a clear list at the end of each chapter of topics covered. I appreciate how Barbori gives a vast number of practical applications for journaling such as increasing confidence, feeling more joy, solving problems, making life decisions, growing as a person, becoming a better writer, and improving overall health and wellness.

I value how Barbori also writes about how journaling can help deal with the painful parts of life, including the losses, griefs, challenges, disappointments, and unrealized dreams.

This book unpacks journaling in ways that really shine a light on how simple it is to do *and* how profoundly it can impact any person who chooses to journal on a regular basis, even for a few minutes each day. The author also covers many other topics as she explores how journaling can be used for one's career, relationships, home, family history, creativity, goals, gardening, homeschooling, learning, faith (there is a chapter on Bible Journaling), and living a grateful life.

The Gift of Journaling is a rich invitation to the page from someone who has benefited greatly from journal writing in her own life. Barbori's passion for the power of journaling is infused in every page and will make you excited to make journaling your own.

As someone who has been journaling and teaching on the life-changing benefits of journaling for decades, as well as leading a global community for journal writers for over seven years, it's a delight to have the fresh and thorough perspective on journaling that this book offers.

I love Barbori's encouragement that journaling can help you reacquaint yourself with who you are. We are living in complex and fast-changing times. Now more than ever, it is important to have tools and practices that can not only ground us but also tune out the noise of the outer world in order to be able to tune into the wisdom and truth of our inner worlds and well-being.

The author shares some of the ways she has used journaling in her own life. This helps readers see how they can use it to great effect in their own lives too. One of the consistent invitations that Barbori makes is the call to come home to the self through journaling. She writes, "Journaling in silence will provide the undivided attention needed to reacquaint yourself with who you are – your likes and dislikes, dreams and goals, thoughts and feelings."

Here's to *The Gift of Journaling: Writing as a Path to Discovery* and how it can guide you to reacquaint you with yourself and this life you are living.

- Lynda Monk, MSW, RSW, CPCC, is the Director of the International Association of Journal Writing. She is passionate about both the transformational power of journaling and the healing benefits of writing in community. She is the co-editor of *The Great Book of Journaling: How Journal Writing Can Support a Life of Wellness, Creativity, Meaning and Purpose* and *Transformational Journaling for Coaches, Therapists and Clients: A Complete Guide to the Benefits of Personal Writing.* She is also the co-author of *Writing Alone Together: Journaling in a Circle of Women for Creativity, Compassion and Connection*. She lives with her family on Salt Spring Island, BC, Canada where she journals almost every day.

Introduction

Welcome! I have been journaling for many years and especially during the past fifteen years, I have seen and known firsthand the benefits of keeping a journal. Some of those benefits that I have found include being able to look back and see the progress I have made in reaching goals, how my goals have changed over the years and decades, and the wisdom I have found to make important decisions through journaling. As I have been on the journey of journaling for many years, I realized that there is much to share about journaling: the joys and benefits, the challenges, the types of journals, and just some of the many resources available.

Why should you journal? Through journaling, you have the perfect place to discover your strengths and weaknesses, likes and dislikes, and gifts and talents. By discovering these things about yourself, you can begin to take the steps to develop them, which can lead to opportunities that otherwise might have passed you by.

Because journaling is different for each journaler, it is best not to compare your time and ability to journal to others'. Journaling will also help you in your own unique way. Here are some of the ways journaling has helped me:

- Writing down the pros and cons of taking a graduate program to decide whether it would help me reach my goals

- Listing fifty types of work I could do to show me the possibilities that could be available
- Jotting the steps I needed to take to publish this book, which resulted in making the process more manageable
- Being able to look back and see the progress I have made in reaching goals
- Seeing how my goals have changed over the years and decades
- Finding wisdom to make important decisions

Part 1 of *The Gift of Journaling* presents the benefits of journaling, creating a journaling routine, overcoming obstacles, and journaling for men while Part 2 goes over the many types of journal to keep and many different topics to write about. In Part 3 of *The Gift of Journaling*, you will find a workbook section. I recommend spending some time going over the questions in this section and when you are ready, write the answers that come to mind. Utilizing the workbook will guide you in creating and sustaining a regular journaling practice.

As you read this book, my goal has been to give you the tools - by sharing how to sustain a journaling routine, overcome obstacles, and providing different types of journals to keep and various topics and questions to journal about - to encourage you to pause, reflect, and get to know yourself better through the practice of journaling. It is my hope that by reading this book, you will gain an appreciation and joy for all that journaling gives and that it will deepen your own regular journaling practice.

Wishing you all the best on your journaling journey,
  Barbori Garnet

Excerpt from the chapter Healthy Home, Healthy You on pages 101-

102 in my book *Home at the Office: Working Remotely as a Way of Life*:

Journal

Writing in a journal on a regular basis — every morning or evening — is an excellent way to destress and get your thoughts down onto paper. There are many benefits to journaling:
- Decreasing stress and anxiety
- Collecting thoughts and practicing fine motor skills
- Writing down goals and noting progress made in achieving them

There are also several types of journals you can keep:

<u>Career/Work Journal:</u> To change careers or find a new or better job, keep a career/work journal. In this journal, you can note things you notice about yourself such as the time of day you work best, the tasks you enjoy doing, whether you prefer working outside, in a home office, or commuting to an office job, and more as you search for, create, and find your ideal remote work or other job position.

<u>Health/Weight Loss Journal:</u> Record your health goals and the steps you are taking each day to achieve them. This can include things such as the foods you eat and when, the quality of your sleep, exercise, and any events in your life which may affect your health like stressful situations (divorce, job loss, conflicts with co-workers, managers, clients or customers, death in the family, unsupportive family members, etc.) or moments to celebrate (new relationship, being debt-free, graduation, etc.).

<u>Money/Finance Journal:</u> Write down your financial goals and track what you do with the money you have, how you spend, save and invest it, and the progress you make to your financial goals.

<u>Dream Journal:</u> This is best done first thing after waking up.

Notice what you dream about and if there are any patterns in your dreams. If you do notice some patterns, you can look into and learn why that might be or what is triggering those images and dreams.

<u>Life Journal:</u> A life journal can be your space to write and remember significant and special moments, days, and events in your life.

<u>Goals Journal:</u> Simply note the goals which you have for various areas of your life — health, money, gardening, travel — and write the things you are doing to reach those goals. For example, if you want to travel somewhere, write down when you want to achieve that, how much you have to save for it, and when you are going to begin booking accommodation — saving information about a romantic inn or a training program presented in a lovely setting/location would support your plans.

<u>Creativity Journal:</u> Explore different ideas, projects, and ways to express and share your creativity. This might mean making a list of creative things you want to try like sculpture, photography, an art class, a new recipe, or even ideas of a better layout for your home office.

<u>Gratitude Journal:</u> Make it a habit to be thankful for what you have and the good things you are blessed with by starting and keeping a gratitude journal. Every morning and/or evening you can make a list of what you are thankful for. It can get your day started off on a positive note or be a perfect winddown at the end of your day.

Select a journal, diary, or notebook that you like and begin to journal and get to know yourself better.

I

Part 1: Create Your Journaling Routine

1

Photo Gallery - Journaling Locations and Tools

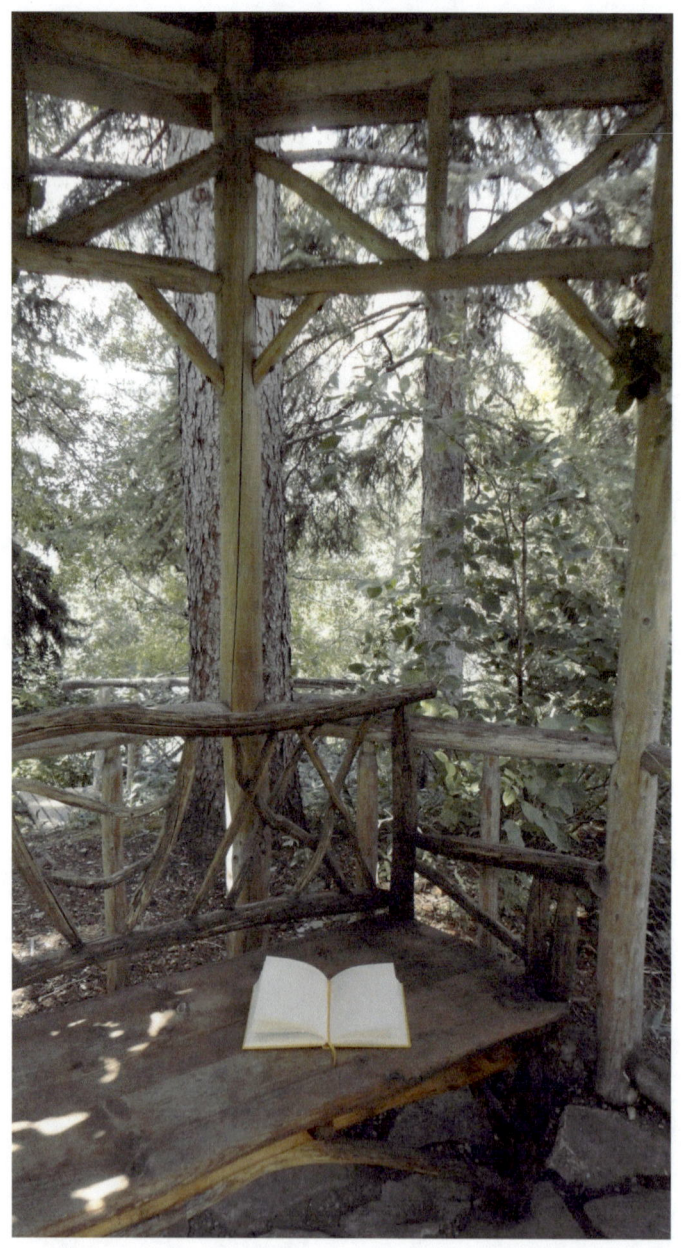

On a sunny and warm day, a gazebo in a garden setting can be an ideal place to journal.

PHOTO GALLERY - JOURNALING LOCATIONS AND TOOLS

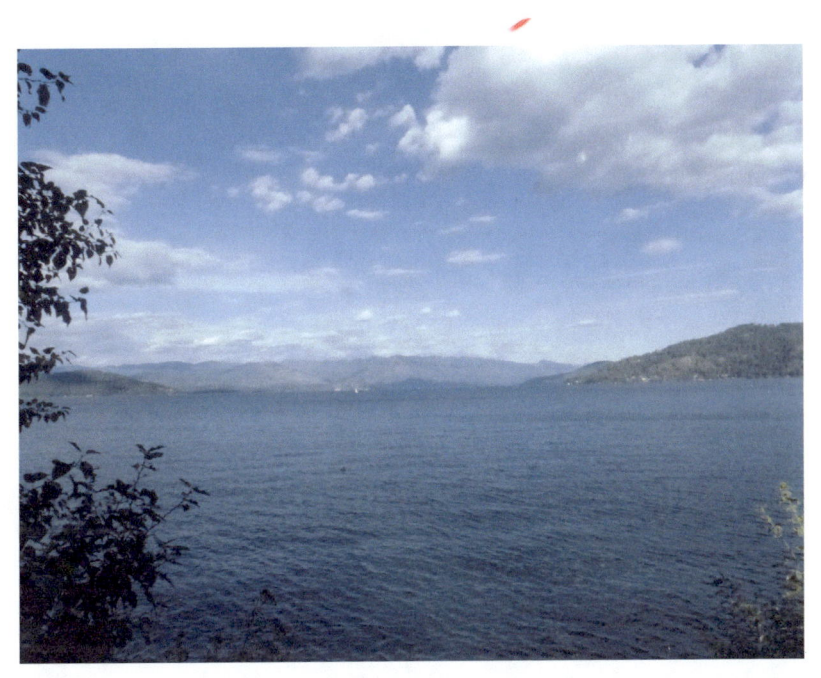

Journaling next to a lake or with a view of a lake can encourage reflection.

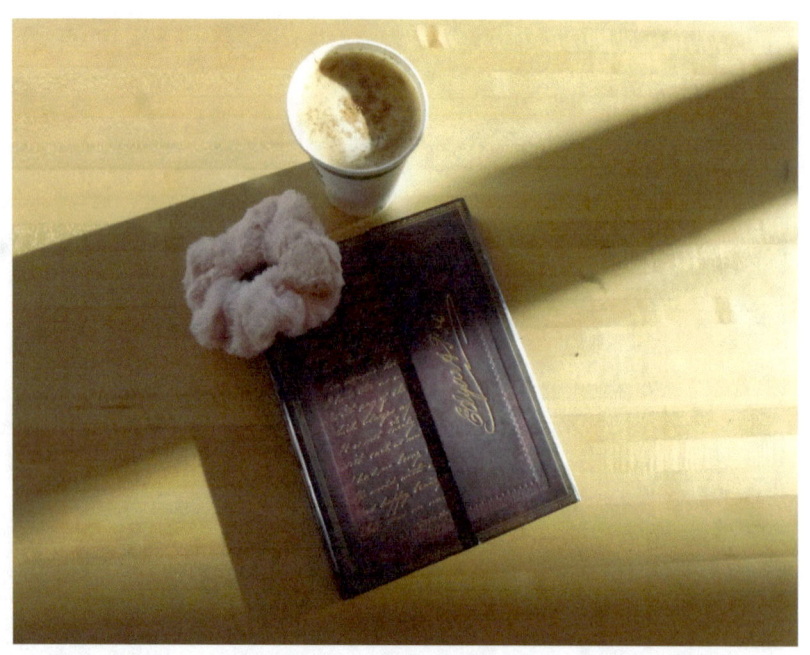

Include a favorite, warm drink - such as tea or cocoa - and something soft - like a blanket or cozy socks - during your journaling time. If writing indoors, find a location where the sun streams in to light the space where you are journaling.

PHOTO GALLERY - JOURNALING LOCATIONS AND TOOLS

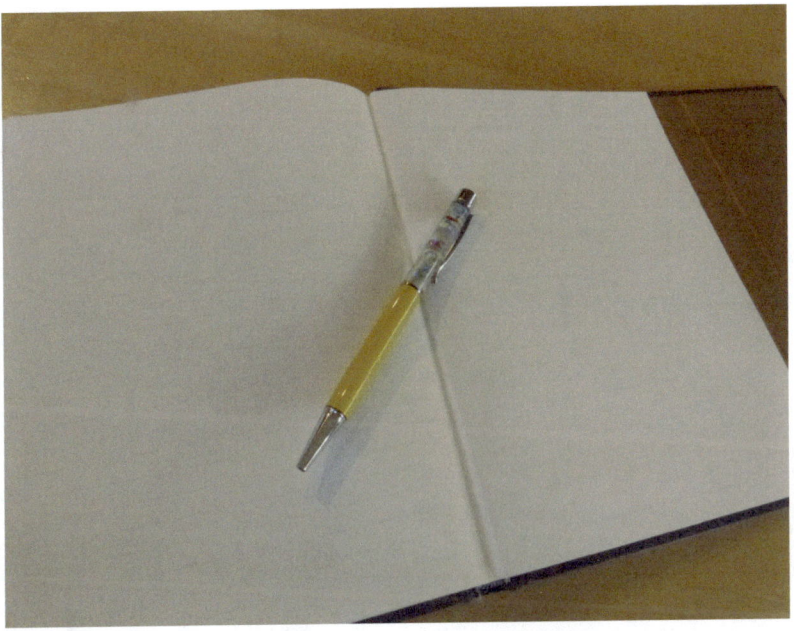

Select a favorite writing tool that is comfortable to hold, easy to write with, and has a cheerful color or pattern.

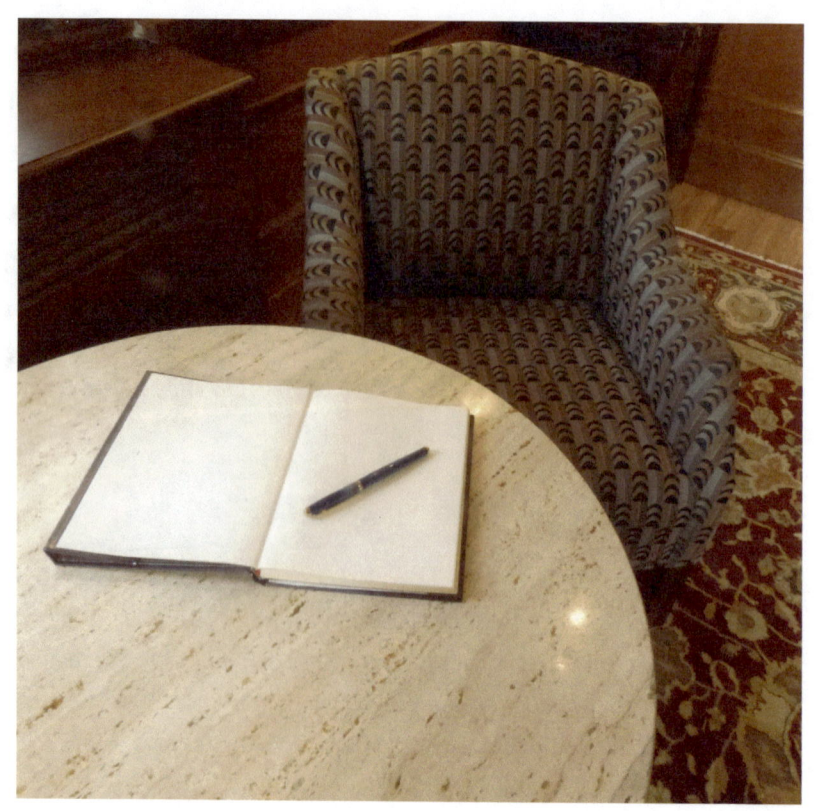

Journaling while seated in a comfortable armchair can help thoughts and ideas flow onto the page.

2

The Benefits of Journaling

"Journal writing is the key to discovering your own unique inner world. Your journal belongs to you. And your journal reflects you. For many journal writers, the journal is also a guide, a map, a treasure trove and a repository of memories."

– Stephanie Dowrick, *Creative Journal Writing*

There are several reasons and benefits as to why someone might want to or choose to journal. In Debbie Travis' book *Joy: Life Lessons from a Tuscan Villa* (Travis, 2021, p. 319), Debbie shares, "Jacky [Brown] tells me science has recognized that journaling – keeping a record of your diet, sleep patterns, habits and goals – is an extremely effective tool. Add five minutes to your bedtime routine and jot down the patterns of your day. This will help you recognize and eventually understand your triggers and your emotional states". With this in mind, this chapter begins with the numerous reasons and benefits of journaling.

Journaling is Portable and Practical
If you are looking for two practical reasons to keep a journal, then these ones are for you:

- Journaling is very portable. You can select a small notebook and pen or pencil that can be tucked away into your pocket or bag and taken with you wherever you go.
- Journaling can easily fit into your schedule. You can write for 5, 15, or 50 minutes each day, thus making it flexible to include in your daily calendar.

Whether you journal while taking the transit to work or during a lunch break, your journal can go with you wherever you happen to be.

Journaling Can Release and Process Emotions and Feelings
An excellent benefit of journaling is that it frees your mind from having to remember things or hold on to emotions. You are able to capture these on paper and then work through and process feelings, emotions, and thoughts at your own pace.

Journaling can be helpful during the following times:

- When experiencing and going through sadness or depression
- Processing and working through grief, whether from the loss of a loved one or perhaps a missed or lost opportunity or time
- Feeling disappointment due to not getting a job offer or promotion that was hoped for, the gradual or definite end of a friendship or relationship, or some other circumstance or event

Journaling Helps Find Answers and Wisdom or Insight
One of my favorite benefits of journaling is the wisdom and insight that can be derived from writing. I have found that many times through journaling about a certain question or difficulty or topic – whether to apply to and pursue a particular degree program, consider the pros and cons of accepting a job offer, the skills and talents that I have and how

I might want to develop them or the ways in which I can use them – the clarity or answer has come during my journaling time. Not only is this a major benefit of and reason to journal but it is also a great feeling and comfort to know that the place in which you journal can be a safe space. It is a place where you can find possibilities, ideas, solutions, opportunities, and answers to questions and problems as well as paths and options for the future.

Your Journal Is Your Best Friend
At times, your journal may be your best friend. When it feels or seems as if no one understands you or as if everything and everyone is changing (moving for jobs, starting new relationships or getting married, starting families, traveling, getting an ideal job or promotion) except you, your journal is always the place you can find openness and comfort in getting down your thoughts (and maybe letting a few tears drop on occasion).

Your journal always has time for you to, well, journal. The page is a listening ear where you can freely share what you are feeling, experiencing, processing, and thinking.

Get to Know Yourself Better and Become Your Own Best Friend
As you begin to journal on a more regular basis, you will notice that you get to know yourself better as well as take the time to think about things that happen. Journaling is a perfect time for this as it provides the necessary quiet for contemplation and reflection.

I suggest that you put all technology away and turn off notifications and sounds if needed. For the first few times, it might be difficult to journal in silence but this can be a good thing to practice and become comfortable with. Journaling in silence will provide the undivided attention needed to reacquaint yourself with who you are – your likes and dislikes, dreams and goals, thoughts and feelings.

Discovering things about yourself leads to growing and learning, which can help you prepare for new paths and opportunities that may come in the future. Learning and discovering about yourself can help increase your self-confidence in your abilities and in your competence to problem-solve or provide solutions for what you should do in the future (take a job, provide a sound answer to a question someone has asked, and more).

Increase Your Self-Confidence
Journaling can increase your self-confidence. How? You will get to know yourself better – what you think, identifying your strengths and struggles or weaknesses, fears, worries and challenges, joys and loves, and your goals. Understanding yourself better will result in knowing what you stand for and believe in and determining the next steps to take to reach goals, thus helping you to walk tall with your shoulders back, head held high, and a smile to greet the world. Expect to increase your self-confidence through journaling on a regular basis.

Adaptable to You Along Your Journaling Journey
While an app or other digital tool might seem easily accessible and convenient and come with customizable options for staying organized and on track with journaling, a journal or notebook is still your best bet because you have access to it at all times.

Unlike the inflexibility of apps and digital tools, here are just a few of the several ways in which a journal or notebook is adaptable and flexible and can change along with you on your journaling journey:

- There are no hidden features or complicated steps to set up

journaling. With a notebook, what you see is what you get.
- You can change back and forth between a smaller or bigger size notebook to fit different sizes of pockets and bags
- Because a journal is analog, you never have to worry about not having a battery or power source to plug in or connect to
- Unless you have a key for locking your journal, you also do not have to worry about remembering a username and password to login to an account before beginning to journal
- Finally, you can take your journals with you wherever you move and you can open up a notebook from five years ago, for example, and see how much you have grown and learned and in what ways your life has changed

How You Live and See Areas of Growth
The more regularly you journal, the more you will be able to look back and see both how you live and the ways you grow over time.

What does it mean, in journaling, to see how you live? It means that you can observe your current habits, patterns, and thoughts to notice if they are helping you improve, reach goals, and stay healthy or whether they are having the opposite effect in your life. Once you truly are aware of how you live, you can begin to identify areas to grow in, decide on changes or actions, and implement them. All of this takes time – seeing how you live and noticing how you grow – so be patient during the process.

Questions, Big and Small
You can ask big and small questions in your journal. For example, if you want to make changes in your life for the better, start by asking small questions and figure out how to answer those by determining small changes you can make today, such as researching gardening

classes, rearranging or organizing a shelf or drawer in your home or office, or starting a website for your new business or hobby. It should be a small and manageable enough task that is easy to complete and gives you a sense of accomplishment first thing in the day.

If you pose big questions in your journal, you might find that they are broad and open-ended. Big questions may be answered or might go unanswered and either way is fine. You might also come back a few days, weeks, or months later and realize that you have an answer to a big question. The point is to ask the question of yourself to ensure that you have given it some thought and are aware of the issue rather than ignoring it or missing it altogether.

Ability to Make Choices
Journaling restores your capability to make choices by listing the pros and cons of jobs to accept, moves to consider, and other decisions to make, noting issues of concern and jotting down things or situations which bother you. Through time, reflection, and discerning your thoughts, feelings, goals, and choices or options, you are better able to make the right or best decisions at the time for yourself as well as be aware of how it would affect those around you.

Once you realize and feel that your ability to make choices has been reawakened and restored, you will feel your self-confidence increase, and new possibilities begin to unfold and open.

A Help in Being Organized
By keeping a journal, or even simply a notebook, you can begin to be more organized. Whether you are a student or parent or you just want to stay on top of work, tracking work-related projects, tasks and assignments, you will notice that your organization increases by

writing down ideas, lists, and things to do. For example, if you are a writer and if you use a journaling method such as Bullet Journaling, creating a Future Log – where you have the next six months divided into squares on the same page – can help you be prepared for article deadlines due in four or five months. I have given the Future Log a try by having the next six months showing on the same page and writing due dates for articles. This helped me to see deadlines at a glance and plan what writing work I needed to do each week or month in order to finish articles and submit them on time.

You can find several examples of and inspiration for creating a Future Log here https://bulletjournal.com/blogs/bulletjournalist/future-log-inspiration/ or take a look at the book *The Bullet Journal Method: Track the Past, Order the Present, Design the Future* by Ryder Carroll. In addition, see chapter **30. Books – on Journaling** for book recommendations related to journaling.

Identifying Priorities
Write down what your priorities are for the month, season or quarter, and year. In my journal, for example, one year I wrote down what my priorities were for the remainder of the summer. By being clear about what my priorities were, I was able to direct my time and energy to the tasks and activities that were important.

Why would you want to bullet your points (list what your priorities are)? First, it can remove the pressure from your mind to have to remember what tasks you need to focus on. This allows your mind to relax and instead redirect the needed energy to what really needs to be done. Second, listing your priorities can help you manage your time to accomplish what is important. Third, you will be able to say "Yes" to things that take precedence or will be a help to what you want to achieve and say "No" to taking on anything else, at least until you check off your priorities or they change in such a way to allow you to start or take on something new.

You can make new lists of priorities as needed or keep a running list and add new items as well as check and cross off things when completed.

Preparing for Detours
On the flip side of writing down your priorities is being prepared for going on detours. Knowing that you will come across side roads as you journal will be a big help to you in staying on track with journaling regularly. These unexpected detours will not throw you for a loop and derail your writing. Instead, they could be a nice, and hopefully, even welcome surprise as they can offer a new chance to pull back the curtain, open the door, and explore some new thoughts, feelings, and possibilities and get to know yourself better.

Examples of journaling detours might include: helping a friend, family member, or neighbor with a move – this could lead to thoughts on considering a move yourself to a preferred location, to be closer to family, or the meaning of home; thoughts on a last-minute summer trip – the excitement of an unexpected trip but the challenge of having to rearrange your schedule; or preparing to start a new job or business in a field that is different from your education – the time commitment and work may both seem daunting. Some of the side roads you will go on in journaling might be quick while others may require more time to fully dive into and write about. This is one of the many gifts of journaling, that it offers and comes with both swift and slow currents of writing time and exploration.

Having the Time to Reflect and Ponder
Time is mentioned often throughout this book. That is because journaling is not to be rushed but instead requires time to be set aside for reflection and pondering.

You may decide to play music in the background while you journal and you can note whether music helps or hinders your writing and reflection. However, you may discover that music might bring up memories, associations, or feelings that have long been buried or hidden but by playing music these are brought to your mind and onto the page.

Improving Health
Many studies have been done over the years which confirm that journaling on a regular basis can improve health by decreasing stress, increasing immunity, and reducing feelings or symptoms of depression, anxiety, and overwhelm. Those who journal regularly may also have increased feelings of well-being, energy, joy, peace, and calm as well as increased confidence in decision-making abilities.

It is important to keep in mind that when journaling, it is best to write about both feelings and thoughts. This means writing down what you are feeling but then going beyond that by trying to make sense of the stress or situation and what you are telling yourself to cope with what is happening. By moving from feelings to thoughts, a journal writer can begin to pick up on patterns, make observations, and set some goals for moving forward.

What is Your Reason to Journal?
A good place to start can be by knowing the reason(s) you want to journal. Knowing this can be a help to staying on track with journaling

on a regular basis. It can also provide direction to how and when you journal or even what resources or inspiration you decide to access to keep you encouraged along your journaling path.

Below are some reasons to journal:

- Begin to understand yourself better
- Improve your writing
- Use your journal as a place to vent and express how you feel and your thoughts about events and situations
- Record your travels
- Help keep you on track with your goals
- Remember your dreams
- Set new plans
- Decide on various actions and directions

What is your reason to journal? One or more from the above list may be your reasons to journal or other reasons might come to mind. Write down your reasons to journal in a place you can refer to so that you can be encouraged and reminded of why to keep journaling.

Keep in mind that journaling is like cross-country running – it requires endurance and strength. Endurance to keep writing on a regular basis and strength to face what may surface as feelings and emotions from what you write on the page. Endurance is one paragraph, one page, one notebook/diary/journal at a time. Strength is continuing to journal even in the face of difficulty or setbacks.

With so many wonderful and varied reasons to begin and continue journaling, let one or more of the reasons in this chapter be the encouragement and inspiration you need to become a journaler. Or, make your own list of why you journal and the benefits of journaling!

The Benefits of Journaling...

- Journaling is Portable and Practical
- Journaling Can Release and Process Emotions and Feelings
- Journaling Helps Find Answers and Wisdom or Insight
- Your Journal Is Your Best Friend
- Get to Know Yourself Better and Become Your Own Best Friend
- Increase Your Self-Confidence
- Adaptable to You Along Your Journaling Journey
- How You Live and See Areas of Growth
- Questions, Big and Small
- Ability to Make Choices
- A Help in Being Organized
- Identifying Priorities
- Preparing for Detours
- Having the Time to Reflect and Ponder
- Improving Health

Notes
Why Write in a Journal and The Benefits of Journaling
1. Travis, Debbie. 2021. *Joy: Life Lessons from a Tuscan Villa.* Random House Canada.
2. *Future Logs.* https://bulletjournal.com/blogs/bulletjournalist/future-log-inspiration/.

3

Create a Routine

"You will never change your life until you change something you do daily. The secret of your success is found in your daily routine."
– John C. Maxwell

The purpose of creating a routine is to have a dedicated time before or after that readies your mind and body for the transition to or from a focused time of writing and back to your day and other tasks that need to be completed. Knowing that you have things that you enjoy and what they are makes it easy to look forward to and easier to do.

Prepare for your journaling session by taking steps to get ready for this time. Things you can do as part of your routine include:

- Making a cup of tea or cocoa
- Reading a few pages from a book
- Going for a walk before beginning to journal
- Putting on a favorite pair of socks
- Wrapping yourself into your favorite blanket
- Running an air diffuser with essential oils

- Sitting in your favorite chair or room
- Playing inspirational background music

These are all ideas to consider implementing as you prepare for journaling. You could also decide to have your routine after you finish journaling and do things such as gentle stretching or playing relaxing music.

Other routines that can quickly become part of your journaling time include:

Practice Handwriting Skills
Journaling can offer a chance to practice handwriting skills. Maybe this will be reason enough to have a regular journaling routine as it might be one of the few times you handwrite and therefore writing becomes a special part of your day.

Practicing handwriting and increasing confidence could lead to developing an interest in improving skills in this area by reading books about or watching video tutorials on calligraphy or taking a calligraphy class or workshop. In addition, honing handwriting skills may result in a desire to write a handwritten letter to a friend or loved one. It is a delight to discover a specially handwritten letter in the mail!

Include Pets
Another suggestion for creating a routine before, after, or while you journal is to use it as a time you spend with your pets. Patting your dog, cat, or other furry friend can be a transition minute or two that helps you prepare to focus on journaling or provides a transition back to the rest of your day. While you journal, your pet can be on your lap or resting by your side. Having your pet close to you can be especially

helpful when what you are writing on the page is sad, difficult, or stressful to journal about. On a lighter note, your pet might also bring to mind fun and special times you want to capture and record in your journal.

Incorporate Water
If the sound of water provides comfort and relaxation to you, try having a water fountain or other water feature on while you journal. The sound of water can be very soothing. Another idea is to have the sound of waves playing as soft background music.

Water can also be refreshing for days when it is hot. If you have the opportunity to journal when you are next to water, such as by a lake, pond, or stream, take advantage of it and note whether writing comes more easily. Visit a park, go to a local beach, take a vacation, or go on a retreat in a location that is close to water or enjoys a view over the water.

Set Aside a Quiet Writing Time for the Entire Family
While you journal, younger kids can work on writing a story of their own and older kids can write in their own journal or work on a school writing assignment. The family writing time can be as short as five to ten minutes long or can be up to thirty minutes long, depending on the age(s) of your child(ren) and independence level and time of day.

You might find that this becomes a new routine for your family that all family members look forward to.

The Routine of Not Having a Routine
Maybe you can write whenever and wherever and so a routine is not necessary to your journaling on a regular basis. That is okay. Instead

of a daily journaling routine, you might prefer to do something special on a weekly or monthly basis. It can be a time to look forward to while at the same time making the routine manageable and scheduling a specific time for it.

Whatever routine you decide to implement, it should be something you enjoy doing and that helps you relax and unwind. You will find that with a little bit of time, your routine will become a welcome habit and a time you look forward to.

Create a routine in your journaling time with these suggestions…

- Practice Handwriting Skills
- Include Pets
- Incorporate Water
- Set Aside a Quiet Writing Time for the Entire Family
- Have the Routine of Not Having a Routine

4

Remember to Make Journaling a Relaxing and Special Time

"Writing opens a part of my mind that experiences meditation and focuses on my own thoughts, feelings, and insights. Writing is intimate, and the smell of fountain pen ink and the feel of smooth paper under the edge of my palm invoke a state of being where I am both reader and writer, questioner and responder."
– Christina Baldwin, *Life's Companion*

Journaling is more than just putting pen to paper to fill the page or the pages of a notebook. Journaling is about a deeper connection to and knowledge of yourself. To make that connection and knowledge happen, journaling needs to be a relaxing and special time . While it need not be a long time set aside to journal, even if it is a short time, it should not be rushed. Instead, it should be a dedicated, uninterrupted five or ten minutes each day during which you journal. To make the most of your time, below are ways to add a touch of relaxation and specialness to those minutes dedicated to journaling.

REMEMBER TO MAKE JOURNALING A RELAXING AND SPECIAL TIME

Collect and Capture the Light
Yes, journaling is a great help to let it all out – tears, frustration, anger, disappointment, sadness, worry, fear, and despair. However, make sure to attempt to capture and collect the light in your life, too – joy, laughter, celebration, love, contentment, hope, dreams, goals, peace, and happiness.

When your journal is filled with light-filled, happy moments and blessings that are sprinkled throughout your days, however small they may seem, it will be more likely that you will like rereading your journals and notebooks in years to come.

Another way to add light to your journaling time is writing during daylight or writing next to a window where natural light comes in. Notice if your energy or focus level or what you journal about is different when you write during daylight or next to or in natural light.

Use an Air Diffuser with Essential Oils
Include the use of a diffuser during your journal writing time. Add 2 to 3 drops of between one to three essential oils to the diffuser. Some suggestions for essential oils to use are:

Relaxing
Lavender
Camomile
Peppermint
Rose

Creativity
Peppermint
Frankincense

Lemon
Lavender

<u>Energizing</u>
Sweet Orange
Peppermint

Select the essential oil depending on the mood you want to be in, whether that is relaxed or energized or something else, and the fragrance you want to enjoy. As you begin to add and use essential oils in a diffuser, you will soon know your favorite combination as well as create new combinations of essential oils that you like.

Light Some Candles
Place and light candles in the location where you will journal. Choose candles that are free of chemicals and made from natural materials – usually candles made from beeswax are the best in this regard though always make sure to check the ingredients. Candles also come in many sizes and fun shapes, like pinecones, bees, flowers and more, giving a touch of playfulness. The light from candles can give the space you are in a warm, inviting light, thus making it more conducive to relaxing and writing.

Personalize Your Journal
Make your journal yours by including those elements that have meaning to you and reflect your personality. Put your own touch and expression in your journal or notebook. There are many ways to do so. Some suggestions and ideas for things you might want to include in your journal are:

- Including quotes from books and songs
- Saving a ticket stub from a concert or performance
- Creating lists
  - Of books you want to read
  - Places you want to travel to
  - 'Top 10', 'Top 50' or 'Top 100' lists of things you want to do or accomplish in life, your dream jobs, favorite books and movies, and more
- Using the Bullet Journal method for one of your journals to learn if you like it and find out if it helps you be more organized and on top of deadlines and assignments
- Letters to yourself and others (but do not send them – they are for you only!)
- Special or memorable letters and postcards you have received from others
- Sketching or drawing plans, dreams, places and locations, or whatever else comes to mind
- Using different colors of ink for different events, feelings, or emotions
- Using different colors of highlighters – yellow, pink, purple, green, or blue – to highlight quotes or phrases that are meaningful or stand out to you in your journal
- Clippings from magazines and/or newspapers
- Artwork and/or photographs
- Alternating between printing and handwriting

While the above may sound a bit like scrapbooking with all the possible items to include, it is meant to show that you can personalize your journal and that no two journals will be alike, not even your own. You can also add a special touch to your journal's cover by enclosing the journal in a specially selected wrap.

Another example of personalization is to use a calendar to keep track of appointments and to paint, draw, sketch, or doodle in your calendar. Or, you can jot notes in a pocket-size notebook when out and about and then transfer to your bigger journal when you are at home.

Notice Voice and Tone
A further way to personalize your journal is to be aware of voice. When a person speaks, they convey a tone and sound of voice. You can do the same in journaling and in other forms of writing (poetry, short stories or fiction, cover letters for job applications, and more). Your choice of words, the length of sentences, and full or abbreviated words all communicate your writing voice and tone.

What are the kinds of voices and tones that can be found in journaling and writing? Below are some emotions or moods that you may pick up on expressed in your own writing or in the writing of others:

- Joy
- Happiness
- Excitement
- Calmness
- Gentleness
- Contentment
- Fear
- Worry
- Sadness
- Anger
- Frustration
- Hurriedness

- Grief
- Disappointment

The voice you write in will change depending on the subject or topic you are writing about and the emotions you feel at the time of writing on the particular topic, event, or experience. Voice can also vary based on the season of life you are in and what you are going through such as whether you are reaching your dreams and goals or feeling unfulfilled in some areas of life.

When you write in your journal on a certain topic or event, make a note to check in about one month later on that same topic or episode. The reason for this is to see if the way you are feeling about the situation has changed due to having worked through feelings related to it, whether solutions to the incident have been found and implemented, or if there are some other grounds for the change in the way you feel.

The use of voice and tone in journaling is another opportunity for you to get to know yourself better by being aware of how you sound and react on the page of your journal. Embrace this time of learning about your voice in the safe and welcoming space of your journal.

Remember the Senses
You have five senses – smell, taste, touch, sight, and hearing. Remember to use them as you describe your feelings, places you have visited, foods you have tried, music you have listened to, and more. These can each infuse more "life" to your journal. Keep in mind, though, that the first priority is to keep on writing rather than stopping frequently to think of the right, fancy word to use or embellishing everything. Why? Stopping frequently can potentially halt the natural, uninhibited, and open flow of your thoughts onto the paper which is what you really

want to capture in the first place.

The Journey of Journaling
The best place to start is to begin by realizing that journaling is a journey. While some journeys have a clear beginning and end, with journaling there is no definite timeline. You can start and finish at whatever time you like. You are never too young or old to embark on the journey of journaling. There will be ebbs and flows to what, where, and how often you journal but that is all part of the path. Take it one day, one page, and one journal or notebook at a time.

Remember, journaling is not a race. Rather, it is a beautiful journey that can last a lifetime, filled with all the welcomed gentle curves and unexpected twists or surprises as you continue a lifelong endeavor of discovery and learning.

Ways to make journaling a relaxing and special time...

- Collect and Capture the Light - Remember to Record Happy, Joyful, Light-filled Times in Your Journal
- Use an Air Diffuser with Essential Oils to Enhance Your Mood
- Light Some Candles
- Personalize Your Journal
- Notice Your Voice and Tone that Shows Through on the Page
- Try to Describe a Variety of Senses in Your Journal Entries
- Remember That Journaling is a Journey

5

Obstacles to Journaling (and How to Minimize or Remove Them)

"Press on. Obstacles are seldom the same size tomorrow as they are today."
– Robert H. Schuller

While there are many benefits to journaling as shared in chapter 2, there can also potentially be several obstacles or challenges encountered either before starting to journal or as one begins to develop and grow a regular journaling practice and routine. Being aware of what those are can help in determining the best solutions and thus steadily continue, at your own pace, on the path of journaling.

Knowing the challenges you may face as you begin, revive, or continue your journey of journaling can assist you in being prepared to find ways to overcome any difficulties along the way. Remember, journaling can be an incredible support to your mental, emotional, and physical health and well-being.

What If You Cannot Journal at Home?
From a lack of privacy to a lack of peace and quiet, there are reasons why it might be necessary to journal in a location away from home. Below are suggestions of places that might be available to you to spend time journaling in that are away from home:

- Coffee shop or café
- Restaurant
- Library
- Retreat centre
- Park, yard, or other outdoor space
- Arts or writing centre or studio
- At work during a lunch or coffee break
- During children's activities or lessons
- Housesitting for someone else while they are away

Do not be discouraged if your living situation is not ideal or conducive to journaling. Instead, take the time to think – and journal – about a solution that will work for you and provide a space that you will look forward to writing in.

Fear and Being Afraid to Journal
You might be feeling fear because of not being sure whether what you would like to journal about is interesting enough or if the writing has spelling and grammar errors. If either or both are the case, my suggestion is to begin with freewriting, meaning writing down on the journal page whatever comes to mind, regardless of correct spelling or grammar. In this way, you get your thoughts on the page without stopping to check whether the topic is interesting or the structure of the sentence is correct. Then, if you feel like it is needed, you can check spelling, grammar, and punctuation rules and apply the lessons

to future journaling.

Another aspect of fear you might feel is related to decision-making. This could be a result of second-guessing yourself in the past, someone else overriding your decisions, or making decisions with some amount of fear based on what-ifs or unknowns. I would encourage you to go to your journal when you need to make decisions so that you can list pros and cons as well as write down potential unknowns and how to address those should they come up. This can assist you to start making decisions with confidence, courage, and conviction.

What If You Want to Journal But Do Not Feel Like It?
If you want to journal but do not feel like it for a day or two or even a few days, then do not force it. It might be that your mind needs to think about and sort through other things or maybe you need to release energy and calm down first before being ready to journal. Or maybe there is a lot going on in your life at the moment. Other things you could do instead of or before journaling are:

- Take a nap
- Take time to stretch
- Listen to music
- Do some other forms of writing (poems, stories, letters)
- Have a cup of tea
- Read a book or magazine
- Listen to an audiobook
- Simply observe and think
- Exercise or move (go for a run, do a yoga class, play basketball, dance, go for a walk)

Try to notice when the times are that you want to journal but do not feel like it. If it happens when there are many changes or life is busy, then schedule it on your calendar to journal for thirty minutes at one point during the week. This way, you are making the commitment to yourself to write down all that is going on. This can help you in two ways – firstly, you can let go of what your mind has been remembering so far and can then focus your energies on other items, and secondly, as you journal, you may come up with new ideas to assist you with current tasks and decisions.

When Is Journaling Helpful?
You might be wondering during what times in life journaling can be helpful. Indeed, there can be many times that journaling is useful, especially ahead of major moments and events. Some of those might include:

- Holidays - To destress, find your centre, and gain clarity and perspective, it can be beneficial to journal ahead of holidays and family visits. You might like to write about your expectations or remind yourself that no matter how busy things get, you will make time each day for self-care and relaxation. This can be one tool to make holidays and family visits less stressful.

- Job Interviews, Other Interviews, and Auditions – Journaling ahead of these moments can assist you in zeroing in on what you want to share about your experience and skills and feel more prepared for the interview. You can also let go of any anxiety or pressure you may be feeling ahead of the interview by writing it down on the page. Finally, a drop or two of a calming essential oil – such as lavender or camomile – on your wrist or temple can help you remain relaxed during the interview or audition.

- Health Concerns and Issues – Writing down what and when you eat, when you go to sleep and wake up and how many hours you sleep, and where pain or other symptoms show up in your body can guide you to make the right decisions for your health. You will be able to have a record where you can review what has been going on and how long you have been feeling a symptom which can then be an aid in relating to a healthcare professional if and when needed.

Sabotaging Your Own Success
If you attempt to begin by self-imposing guidelines or rules that are not realistic for what you can commit to, then you risk setting yourself up for disappointment, failure, or both, and potentially sabotaging any success you might have had.

To help ensure success, start with what will be manageable for you as well as what you will like. Perhaps it means journaling every second day – and writing a short paragraph – rather than every day. Or journaling once a week on the weekend – and writing one or two pages – so that it fits with your schedule and that you look forward to and enjoy it. Take the small, manageable steps you need to guarantee your success.

When Life Is Too Overwhelming
By beginning to journal, or journaling regularly, what surfaces on the page may make you feel overwhelmed. If that occurs, proceed at a pace that you feel comfortable with.

It can also happen that when life is too overwhelming and one is crying often, that it can be hard to journal regularly because writing can bring up the same emotions and feelings all over again.

However, I highly encourage you to continue journaling regularly even when you are feeling so many emotions and life is overwhelming. But instead of doing too much, write only one sentence or one short paragraph every day or two. The reasons for keeping on journaling are to:

1) Find your centre, solace, grounding, and comforting place in your journal
2) Be able to look back on this time and recognize how much inner strength you have, how much you have learned, and how much you have grown. That will be worth acknowledging, celebrating, and being proud of.

Facing Disappointment
Disappointment or other feelings such as failure, sadness, discouragement, or disinterest in life can each impede or hinder one's ability to journal. When these feelings are present in an overwhelming proportion, it is important to realize and remember that journaling is only one of the tools available to help you process, heal, and move forward in what you are feeling. Some other modalities that may assist you include guided imagery, massage or self-massage, counseling or therapy, spending time in a garden or in nature, or going on a retreat.

Coping Mechanism
One important thing to know about journaling is that in some instances or circumstances, journaling could be more of a coping mechanism.

For example, a journaler may feel that moving to a different residence or home, neighborhood, or city would help to solve some issues or be able to move forward in life. However, family obligations or financial situations – lack of income, needing to start or grow a business, needing a job, needing a higher income, or having debt – may be in the way of moving or making a change.

This is where it is helpful to realize that journaling may be a great coping mechanism or tool while in the situation rather than the actual tool used to make the change. Journaling can help you make your way day by day and be a place to write down thoughts or future action steps to take even if change is not possible or feasible right away.

Feeling Stuck
If you feel stuck in your life, use your journal to help you move through this time. Feeling stuck can relate to many areas:

- Stuck on a creative project or in a creative rut
- Stuck or stagnant in a relationship (personal, business, etc.)
- Stuck on what to do or what your mission or purpose is in life
- Stuck by not having fulfilled goals or dreams from earlier times or seasons in life and not sure how to move forward

Remember that it might take a bit of time to sort and work through being stuck. You might need other supports and resources – spending time in nature, seeing a therapist, working with a career or life coach, going on a retreat, or reading a book. Make sure to have your journal with you to record insights, ideas, and action steps that come when interacting with a support or resource or simply journal on your own.

Not Always the Answer
Sometimes, journaling will not be the only answer to expressing or processing how you feel or the emotions you feel. When those times come, do what you need to do to release negative thoughts and emotions – cry, scream or shout (make sure there is not anyone

close by or you might scare them which is not what you want to do or have happen), go for a run, do a workout or even a few stretches, sing along with a song, or simply lie quietly in a calm and relaxing space or environment, take a nap or go to sleep, or just think and let your thoughts drift and wander. In addition to journaling, find other healthy avenues through which to express what you feel to begin finding answers and solutions to help you move forward.

Taking a Risk
By journaling, what are you taking a risk on learning, discovering, and knowing about yourself that you might or might not like? Can you take the risk of not learning something new, in case you do not like it?

Journaling can be and is a risk. You are opening your heart, peeling it back layer by layer.

By starting or resuming journaling, potential obstacles encountered may include:

- Not Being Able to Journal at Home
- Feeling Fear
- Not Feeling Like Journaling
- Not Sure of When Journaling is Helpful
- Sabotaging Your Own Success
- Being Overwhelmed in Life
- Facing Disappointment
- Using Journaling as a Coping Mechanism
- Feeling Stuck
- That Journaling is Not Always the Answer
- Taking a Risk on Learning About Yourself

OBSTACLES TO JOURNALING (AND HOW TO MINIMIZE OR REMOVE THEM)

Do you face any of the above obstacles or are there other issues or hindrances that you might come across when it comes to journaling? Realizing that there are things that may come up along your journey is the first step to being prepared and then determining the best way to work through the obstacles with support in place, tools at hand, and at the right pace for you.

6

Being Part of a Community and Finding Support

"Community is about finding people that share the same vision as you."
– Anonymous

Journaling can include being part of a community and finding resources and support to assist you to grow in journaling, reaching journaling goals, and being encouraged to continue journaling in the face of discouragement or obstacles. Below are some suggestions and ideas for places and ways to find the community, support, and inspiration you may need.

Community
For some, finding and being part of a local or an online community can help to be more consistent with journaling. This does not mean that you need to or should feel compelled to share anything – not even one sentence – from your journal. Rather, being part of a group of writers and journalers can help with accountability for staying on track to journal regularly.

Journal Memoirs
It can help to read the journals of others, whether contemporary journal writers or journal writers from the past, even from previous centuries. Some suggestions include:

- *The Journal Keeper: A Memoir* by Phyllis Theroux
- *Roughing It in the Bush* by Susanna Moodie
- *Her Life, Letters, and Journals* by Louisa May Alcott
- Journals by Winston Churchill, Henry David Thoreau, and others

The above are included in chapter **30. Books - Journal Memoirs (Journals Written by Others)**. By reading others' journals, you will learn that people have experienced challenges that might be similar to what you are going through or that others have different insights and thoughts on situations that will provide you with perspective, hope, and new ideas.

You will also see that each journal writer has a unique style of writing and expressing what they are thinking and going through. This can give inspiration for topics and feelings you might want to write about or questions you might want to ask and address in your journal, either now or to make a note to come back to it later.

Books and Articles
In chapter **30. Books - on Journaling**, you will find recommendations for books on journaling such as:

- *Creative Journal Writing: The Art and Heart of Reflection* by Stephanie Dowrick
- *Journal to the Self: Twenty-Two Paths to Personal Growth* by Kathleen Adams, M.A.

- *Life's Companion: Journal Writing as a Spiritual Practice* by Christina Baldwin
- *100% Happiness: A Guided Journal to Enhance Your Daily Life* by Raphaelle Giordano

If you are looking for new prompts or ideas to infuse into your journaling routine, these can be a great source of inspiration.

You can also search online for articles about journaling and on topics such as health benefits of journaling, journaling prompts, types of journals, how to make your own journal, and more. See what interests you and take it from there.

Courses
There are courses, classes, and workshops that you can take to expand your skills and confidence in journaling. If you attend or take a class, you will leave feeling inspired and will have met several people who also have an interest in journaling. Be open to what the presenter shares and apply the tips and techniques that would be most beneficial to your journey.

Journaling can be a time of connecting, learning, and growing, both on your own and with other journalers and writers. Take the time to discover the community, resources, and support that are the right fit for you by considering these suggestions:

- Joining a Local or Online Community
- Reading Journals by Contemporary and Historic Journal Writers
- Finding Books and Articles on Journaling
- Taking Courses

7

Journaling - For Men

"A man lives by what he believes in."
– Emmett Ryker in *The Virginian* (TV Series)

"The real man smiles in trouble, gathers strength from distress, and grows brave by reflection."
– Thomas Paine

Is Journaling for Men?

Journaling can be an excellent tool to reflect on areas in a man's life to improve and help a man sort through information ahead of making choices. Through journaling, men can increase confidence in their communication skills, gain the strength and courage needed to make and act on decisions, and more.

Tips for Men to Journal

Here are a few tips for men to assist them in their journaling practice:

- Use point form to jot down thoughts if that works better and is more efficient for you
- Make journaling part of your morning routine – after you wake up or before going to the gym – or evening routine – after finishing at the gym or before bed
- Journal to find solutions, discern feelings, or list ideas or plans for the future

Understanding a Man's Roles and Responsibilities
What roles do you have in life? Are you a husband, father, son, brother, uncle, nephew, and/or cousin in your family? Are you a manager, owner, employee, colleague, neighbor, volunteer, etc. in your work, church, and community life? Knowing the important roles you have in life, and how you carry out those roles as well as the effect and influence your behavior, attitude, and decision-making have on others, can help you begin to identify areas that need improvement.

Your responsibilities may include:

- Showing up to work on time
- Doing your best at work
- Leading and managing employees at work
- Maintaining/improving/upgrading your home and yard
- Loving, leading, protecting, and providing for your wife and children
- Dropping off and picking up your kids from school and activities
- Having a budget and planning financially for the future

To better understand a man's roles and responsibilities in life, here are recommended resources to read and study:

- *The 7 Habits of Highly Effective People* by Stephen Covey
- *What's the Difference?: Manhood and Womanhood Defined According to the Bible* by John Piper
- *The Resolution for Men* by Stephen Kendrick and Alex Kendrick

Developing Character
You can make lists of characters in movies and books whose character you would like to emulate or whose actions show courage, conviction, bravery, honesty, self-confidence, humility, etc. You can list your childhood heroes and those you look up to as an adult. You might also like to make a note of what you were going through at the time to identify what traits your heroes possessed or which circumstances they found themselves in that you connected with.

Making Decisions
Both at work and at home, men regularly have to make decisions for themselves, their families, and/or their employees. Journaling is a great way for men to clarify their thoughts as they sort through various options and make a choice. Decisions may require many considerations such as:

- Practical implications – consequences, delays, goals, vision, plans, impressions/images, etc.
- Emotional underpinnings or reactions – reactive or preventive, positive or negative
- Moral and/or ethical standards – of the business world, company, society, family of origin, own family (wife and children), or friends

Many times, making a decision might not seem easy or straightforward as there can be nuances – consequences, details, plans/goals to achieve, or suggestions while upholding personal standards – to consider.

For example, decisions you might encounter that include practical, emotional, and moral/ethical reasons could be:

a) Whether you should disclose problems on an old vehicle you want to sell quickly or put some time and a little bit of money to fix the vehicle and sell it at a better price
b) If you should take a job that pays well, as your family could use the additional income, but would require longer work hours or commute taking you away from your family or instead put the time into starting your own side business to bring in the needed income
c) Whether you should take a well-paying job that requires you to follow a health policy or order you do not feel good about following or perhaps consider looking for a lower-paid job aligning with your values and renting out part of your home to bring in additional income
d) If you should buy a new fancy car so that you would look successful to family, friends, and neighbors but this purchase would place your family into debt for a longer period of time or drive a kind of vehicle not suitable for family lifestyle. There may be alternative solutions one could write in the journal such as renting the car of your dreams for a get-away-weekend with your wife or even a test drive of the desired model.

As you take into account the different aspects of choices, it is just as important to consider whether you would feel good about yourself in making a choice. Listing the reasons for making a decision can help men stand strong in their determination or conviction, knowing that what they are standing for is the right thing to do.

The other side of this is to write or journal about why it is difficult to make some decisions. Some reasons could be:

- Encountering an emotional basis underlying the issue
- Identifying emotional reluctance to address an issue
- Other people's reactions to the decisions you make
- The effect of decisions made by you on others

In your journal, determine the whys behind the reason so that you can take action to then make the needed decision for yourself and those in your care. If you are wondering whether you are making the best or correct decision, there are a few things to keep in mind:

1) What is best or correct for you and/or your family may look different from what is best or correct for another man and/or his family
2) Even if the decision is hard to make and might result in unfavorable circumstances or situations for you and your family, there should be certain principles that are non-negotiable such as speaking the truth (in a firm but kind manner), doing good, being respectful, and being wise in the use of money and time

Improving Communication
Communication is essential in daily life, personal relationships, and business interactions. Journaling is an excellent tool to help men understand and work on as well as perfect their communication skills. Give journaling a try to assist you to clarify your thoughts.

Use regular journaling times to enhance your communication skills by:

- Noting topics or subjects that are more difficult, awkward, or uncomfortable to bring up or talk about with others. For example, are these topics difficult to address because your family did not discuss them growing up? Begin to identify these memories to see

patterns and take the steps necessary to work on overcoming any hesitation.
- Writing down the points you would like to address when speaking with others
- Writing down the solutions or changes you would like to see:
  - Implemented at work or in your business
  - Made at home or in personal relationships
  - Take place in your life
- Recording your feelings, emotions, or reactions about something that has happened or what someone said. Give some thought to whether the way you are reacting is how you observed your father or other father-figure reacting in a similar situation to understand why you might be reacting in a similar way.

While addressing the above communication areas in your journal, keep in mind that you do not need to use full sentences – instead, you can use point form to jot down thoughts if that works better for you.

Working on Relationships
Have you noticed that relationships with your wife, children, other family members, or friends have become more distant? Do you find that you do not know the likes, dislikes, plans, and goals of close family? If any of these are relatable, take to your journal to improve your relationships by:

- Writing down questions to ask loved ones about their likes, dislikes, plans, and goals and record what you learn so that you review it and check in with loved ones on a regular basis on the things that are important to them
- Jotting down ideas for ways to spend quality time with your wife, kids, other family members, and friends

- Making note of things family members and friends say that they would like to do and that are meaningful and special to them

As you begin to notice the little and big things that are important to loved ones and employ your journal to assist you in remembering and applying meaningful connections, conversations, and actions, you will start to see these relationships grow closer and know these special people in your life better.

Keeping Track of To-Do Lists
Whether it is a 'Work', 'Honey-Do', or 'Home Projects' to-do list, a journal is an excellent place to keep these lists. You can keep each of these lists in one journal, making them easy to find and access, and easily started, added to, and finished. If you are looking for something to do in the evenings after work or on the weekends, refer to the lists you have made and see what you could spend some time on so that it is completed sooner for your and your family's enjoyment.

Making New Friends and Growing Long-Time Friendships
Whether a man already has many friends or is looking to increase his social circle, continuing to journal regardless of the number of people in a man's social network is important. Why?

If a man wants to meet and make new friends – whether because of moving to a new city, entering a different life stage, developing new interests, or for other reasons – keeping a journal can be a helpful support. In a journal, you can:

- Brainstorm ideas and ways to meet friends
- List the qualities that make for a good friend and friendship
- Write down the qualities that would make you a good friend to

others and the areas you need to work on to become a better friend

For a man who has many new and long-time friends, a journal can be a great place to record the good times and memories made with friends. Being able to recall the adventures enjoyed with friends can be a fun time down memory lane. A journal can also be used to capture ideas for future activities to do with friends such as camping and/or hiking trips, father/son outings, picnics, or outdoor skills.

Finding Strength, Support, and Courage
If you are facing a tough decision or challenging time in life, refer to your journal to look back on other difficult circumstances that you have overcome in the past. This can assist in reminding you that you have the strength and courage needed to face what is in front of you now. Looking back in your journal on other decisions you have made can also help you recall how you made choices in the past – whom you asked or where you turned for advice, if you listed pros and cons to a situation, if conditions are still the same or if they had changed, or how you organized your thoughts.

Journaling can be a tool for men to use to assist them in clarifying actions and beliefs. These are the ways that journaling can help:

- Understanding a Man's Roles and Responsibilities
- Developing Character
- Making Decisions
- Improving Communication Skills
- Working on Relationships
- Keeping Track of To-Do Lists
- Making New Friends and Growing Long-Time Friendships
- Finding Strength, Support, and Courage

8

Journaling Through...

> "To everything there is a season, A time for every purpose under heaven:"
> – Ecclesiastes 3:1 (KJV)

...the Changes

Sometimes, it feels that change is the only constant in life. And while it is true that life is always filled with changes, there can be times when it seems there are more changes than usual or that one feels like one can handle.

When changes come, begin by acknowledging how you are feeling – overwhelmed, relieved, fearful, apprehensive, excited, or something else – and then see how the shift opens up or allows for a new possibility or opportunity. This happened to me one spring – in my work life, there were many changes at work which included working hours, colleagues, and the direction of the company I worked for. Once I knew that definite decisions had been made by the business owner with regard to these work changes, I had more confidence. New opportunities opened up including increased time to work on my writing projects, availability for other contract work, and time and energy to consider and apply for other positions as well as plan a couple of road trips.

It is also good to consider what you can manage during periods of many shifts. For instance, with lots of changes going on at work or in your personal life, you might decide that it is best not to take on anything new in other areas of your life. Or, if there are lots of changes at work during the week, try to schedule only one big thing on the weekend to give yourself time to rest as well as contemplate.

Remember that change is part of life and also that change can bring certainty by knowing a decision or shift has been made definitely one way or another. Your journal is there to support you during life's changes by:

- Revealing opportunities
- Jotting down options
- Describing emotions
    - I am afraid that "x" will happen. If it happens, I can do…
    - I am excited because these opportunities will open…
    - I am overwhelmed. What can I do to reduce the sense of being overwhelmed? What can I do to prepare for future situations?

…the Joys and Laughter
It is wonderful to be able to write about the laughter we share with loved ones, the times we celebrate the accomplishments of friends, and the myriad of ways that joy shows up and is a blessing in our everyday lives. Take the time to note the variety of manners and activities that joy, laughter, love, and more are gifted to you:

- Flowers delivered to your door from friends or family
- Coffeehouse visit or afternoon tea with a friend
- Dinner out to celebrate a milestone or accomplishment
- Enjoying perfect weather while strolling through a park and having ice cream
- Playing music with a group of friends
- Singing while washing dishes or preparing dinner (find a YouTube playlist of your favorite songs)

There are countless ways that we are blessed with joy, laughter, happiness, and love in life. Make sure to include these moments in your journal.

...the Challenges
By writing about the challenges that you are going through, you will later be able to look back and see how you overcame them:

- Maybe you took things one hour or one day at a time
- Perhaps you spent more time relaxing and minimizing stress
- Or maybe you thought of new solutions to solve the problem or challenge that had come up
- Perhaps you reached out to people who responded or someone reached out to you for support, and you were able to help and that allowed you to see your own situation from a new perspective

Whatever difficulty you have faced, currently face, or will face in the future, continue to journal through those times. Journaling will help to see you through and will remind you that you do have options and can think of solutions to implement successfully.

...the Adventures

Life is filled with adventure! Whether it is the adventure of love, hiking and spending time outdoors, or launching a business, there is always an experience, quest, or feat that can be thrilling. By choosing to capture these occurrences, you will remember and begin to see that your life is filled with one adventure after another. You can keep mementos – a theatre ticket, a bookmark, a business card, a photo, or magazine clippings – to remind you of the experience.

...the Seasons of the Year

Journaling is an activity that can be done the entire year through – winter, spring, summer, and fall. It can be adapted to the changing of the year's seasons. When the light is out earlier in the morning and later at night, you might find that you prefer to journal at a different time.

You might discover that you prefer to write or journal at a different time of day or a different spot or place – armchair, desk, porch or deck, etc. – depending on the season. Perhaps the way the sun falls on a chair or on the porch is perfect in the summer and the couch by the fireplace is the ideal spot during the winter.

As you begin, grow, and develop your journal routine, I recommend at least including the date with each entry. Why? It can be interesting to look back and note during which months or seasons you do more writing. For example, you might discover that you journal quite frequently and on a regular basis during the winter and summer seasons. The reason for this could be that when the nights are dark and long in the winter, it is soothing to sit in a favorite chair or nook or on the bed and journal. In the summer, with the warmer weather and daylight longer, it can be delightful to linger outside on a porch or in the yard or in a park and journal to one's heart's content. Begin to observe these things with the change of seasons and whether you write more or less at different times of the year.

...the Seasons of Life
Another side to journaling through the seasons is that of writing through the seasons – or stages – of life. To cope with the demands, challenges, and joys of raising a family, you might find that you journal more often during this season and time of life. Or maybe the opposite is true – you only have five minutes here and there to spend time journaling. Other examples of seasons of life and life stages include:

- First or new job
- Post-secondary (college, university, trade school)
- Newlywed
- New parent
- Empty nest
- Retirement
- Widowhood

Some seasons of life might include both a change in life stage as well as other accompanying changes. For example, the new life stage of being a newlywed might come not only with being newly married but also with a move to a new home in a new location which is another change in itself.

Which season do you find yourself in now or about to begin? Do you find it a struggle to balance the stage of life you are currently in with the stage of life a family member – such as a parent or grandparent – is in? How do these different life seasons affect when or how often you journal?

Are there other life stages you can think of? Some seasons of life may stay for shorter or longer periods of time, or come earlier or later or may not come, but it is important to realize that seasons are always changing. Try to be thankful for and capture the blessings and joys that are to be found throughout the different times and stages of life.

Remember to journal through…

- The Changes
- The Joys and Laughter
- The Challenges
- The Adventures
- The Seasons of the Year
- The Seasons of Life

9

Journaling Do's and Don'ts

As **Part 1: Create Your Journaling Routine** of this book comes to a close and before beginning **Part 2: Types of Journals**, here are a few guidelines to keep in mind as you journal:

- Do write in your journal on a regular basis – daily in the morning or evening, every two or three days, weekly, or monthly
- Do date your entries. At the very least, write down the month and year if not the actual day. You will be able to look back and see whether you were going through a time of quiet and calm or busyness, of joy or sorrow, or of melancholy or reflection.
- Do try new ways of journaling – dot journaling, making lists, etc.
- Do be creative in your journal – sketch or draw, paint, write poems, draft letters, scrapbook photos, tape ticket stubs, and more
- Don't limit yourself or place any limits on or box yourself in when it comes to journaling style or types of journals
- Don't worry or be concerned about what or how you write. Instead, write down as many thoughts that come to mind, including ideas, plans, goals, places to visit, books to read and movies to watch, conversations you had or want to have, and more.

# II

Part 2: Types of Journals

*In this part of The Gift of Journaling, we will explore 15 types of journals and their focus. As you read and decide on what to address in your journal, you may realize that you want to combine some—such as **Career/Work/Business Journal** and **Money/Finance Journal**, for instance—and that is okay. You can select a different journal or notebook for each theme or choose a notebook that already is divided into sections to make journaling more manageable and have everything in one place.*

10

Career/Work/Business Journal

"Do what you can with all you have, wherever you are."
– Theodore Roosevelt

In my book, *Home at the Office: Working Remotely as a Way of Life* (Garnet, 2021, p. 101), I wrote, "To change careers or find a new or better job, keep a career/work journal. In this journal, you can note things you notice about yourself such as the time of day you work best, the tasks you enjoy doing, whether you prefer working outside, in a home office, or commuting to an office job, and more as you search for, create, and find your ideal remote work or other job position."

Through the many demands and changes you will experience during your career and working years, your **Career/Work/Business Journal** can be your constant companion. Whether you are excited about a job promotion or bonus or disappointed by a negative job review or interaction with a client or colleague, your journal is the place to go to when you need to clarify what you are feeling and the direction you are going in. Below are some pointers for areas to journal on to help you prepare for opportunities, make changes in your work, and grow in your career.

Prepare for Interviews
A **Career/Work/Business Journal** can be used to assist you in preparing for job interviews. Ways to do this include:

- Writing out your answers to potential interview questions
- Making a list of questions – such as about the role, tasks, responsibilities, hours, and company – to ask during the interview
- Listing ways to stay calm during an interview such as by taking deep breaths before the interview starts, feeling confident, and knowing that you are prepared

After the interview concludes, you may like to return to your journal to write down how the interview went, how you feel (happy, relieved, nervous, etc.), and if you could have answered questions differently. This can be a great way to pause and reflect on an interview and then be able to move on and prepare for other job applications, upcoming interviews, or new opportunities.

In addition, consider using your journal to help you get ready for other types of interviews. For example, if you are a writer who interviews others, you can write down your list of questions for interviewees. Or, you might jot questions and notes ahead of board interviews, list what to prepare for auditions, or make note of what to expect in phone, video, group, panel, or lunch or dinner interviews.

Consider Working from Home
As you go through the different stages of life, the when and where of work might change. In your **Career Journal**, you may wish to explore the possibility of working from home - it could be the solution to

being at home while your children are young or being able to travel on the road for an extended length of time or fulfilling your wish to be in control of your schedule for the day.

While considering the option of remote work, use your journal as a space to ponder ideas such as what type of work-from-home business or remote work you could do. Could you work on contract, start your own business, or continue to work for your current employer while transitioning to working remotely? Also give some thought to what hours would be a good fit with your schedule, responsibilities, priorities, plans, and both personal and financial goals. In addition to the positive aspects of working remotely, you can address any potential obstacles or challenges you might encounter and brainstorm ideas to minimize or eliminate them.

To learn more about and consider the possibilities available in working from home, make sure to read my book *Home at the Office: Working Remotely as a Way of Life*.

Explore the Option of Hiring a Career or Business Coach
If you want to grow and expand your business or change careers, you could journal about whether you need to hire and work with a career or business coach. You can begin by listing the areas in which you need help in order to see new growth. Listing the areas can assist you in determining which career or business coach might be right for you and gaining clarity on the direction you want to go.

Give Drawing a Try
Your journal can be a space for not only writing but also drawing about work. You could draw what your ideal office space would look like and how it would be organized and decorated, draw product sketches or

diagrams, or design mock-ups of and sketch logo ideas. These, in turn, might inspire you to make small changes – such as painting the walls a different color, adding a mirror to seemingly make the space bigger, hanging artwork to enliven the space, or changing the height of your table or chair – to your current workspace to make it more conducive to getting work done or perhaps lead to the development of new products. Remember that in chapter **2. The Benefits of Journaling**, we explored that journaling gives you the ability to find answers and make choices.

Discover Your Gifts and Talents
A benefit of keeping this type of journal is that you begin to notice and learn the gifts, talents, and skills you have been given. By developing your gifts, new doors may open that you might not have thought possible and you will have the chance to make a positive difference in the lives of others. This can be an encouragement and can assist in knowing which path to take to both use your skills and reach goals.

Capture Entrepreneurial Ideas
This type of journal can be an excellent support to journalers whether they are starting a new or another business or adding new offerings to their current business. Use your journal to both record ideas you think of and refer back to ideas that merit further development.

Ideas that may come can be for businesses that offer products, services, or both and for businesses that are in a brick-and-mortar location, online, or some combination thereof. Make sketches of logos, designs and products, determine pricings, and more. Is there a product or service that is missing or could be delivered to customers in a better, more efficient or unique way? An **Entrepreneurship Journal** can be the perfect place to brainstorm ideas and record things you see that work well or make note of where improvement is needed. You can also cover to-do items and tasks such as due dates or filings for business taxes, business license renewal, website domain renewal, and other annual events.

This type of journal can work well for both new and established businesses, providing a framework for new businesses or new guidance and vitality for established businesses. For instance, you can take your journal with you when you are out and about, for example at a business conference or trade show, so that when you come across a product or service similar to what you are developing, you can jot down right away the price of the item or any interesting features. When you are close to launching or releasing your product, refer back to your journal to see the price range and then determine where yours fits in while remembering that there are a variety of factors that go into deciding on a price: product features and complexity, cost and availability of materials, the time and skill to make the product or provide the service, market demand, profit margin, and other aspects or considerations.

You can also use the journal to reflect on which tasks you like to do, when it might be time to hire help and for which tasks, and what you would look for to contract, delegate to, or partner with someone else to complete a job.

Consider Technology
Keeping notes of steps for transferring, saving or downloading files, where files are located or saved, keyboard shortcuts, what you did to reboot your computer last time, how to check security and anti-virus software, and more can be a huge help to save time in the future when the same action is needed. You can also write down the names of software and programs that would be helpful to you in your current

or future job, the features you would like in your next computer or camera, and models of computers or cameras you are considering for your next purchase.

Your Career – Blazing Your Own Trail or Following In Someone Else's Footsteps?

Have you made your own decisions regarding career choices or have you been following in someone else's footsteps? Did you have any guidance from parents, extended family members, teachers, professors, counselors, friends, or others in helping you determine what education and career choice would suit your interests, goals, and plans for the future? We may have intended to choose a different career that aligned better with our gifts and talents. However, because of family expectations or traditions or the family business, these can affect why we chose a certain major or degree in post-secondary, what career we worked in, and where we lived. Sometimes the family attitudes or expectations and the reason for them (e.g., financial security, responsibility, respect for the profession or position, or maybe freedom, etc.) are unspoken or buried deep down, and writing them in the journal enables you to examine them if they still apply or if one's gifts or plans are better or more closely aligned with one's goals and vision for the future.

Other things to give some thought to are whether career choice and pursuit of a career were valued in your family as being important for both boys and girls and if you were encouraged to learn and excel and do your best to achieve or if the opposite was true. You may also realize you were expected to follow in a family member's footsteps such as studying to become a lawyer, doctor, engineer, or other profession or trade.

Identify Negative or Toxic Work Environments

In your **Career/Work/Business Journal**, you may also decide to record and write about instances of a toxic work environment. Why? First, it can help you manage stress and emotions that surface as a result of bad experiences at work. Second, and just as important, it can assist you in clearly identifying the toxic behaviors and patterns encountered as well as steps to take to remove yourself from the situation. For example, the negativity might stem from colleagues, management, or clients or customers. Once you have identified the areas that are causing problems, you can then determine whether to:

- Bring it to the attention of management and see if changes can be made in the company
- Switch to a different department within the company
- Leave the company and find a job at a different company in the same city or move elsewhere for a new job
- Start a new business with a different focus so as to be working with a different group of clients or customers
- Find another solution that would work better

If you find yourself in a toxic work environment, make notes in your journal about your health on a daily basis and record any changes you notice, feel, or experience. Examples would be trouble falling asleep or staying asleep, changes in appetite, gaining weight, increased cravings, and decreased motivation to exercise or go to work. Do the best you can to mitigate and minimize negative health effects while at the same time doing your best to change your work situation for the better.

To assist during a time of being in a toxic work environment, here are some questions to address in your journal:

- Are there others who this problem is affecting? If yes, who and where are they, and how is the situation affecting them?
- Am I in a position to resolve the problem?
- Do I have the skills to resolve this problem?
- Am I willing to deal with the problem? If not, why not?
- If the problem is something I cannot resolve myself, who can? What is the chain of command? Who do I have the best rapport with? How do I describe the concern (tone of voice, choice of words, etc.)? What can I do to inform them of the problem and what documentation do I need to provide or share with them? What can I do to help them make things better?
- What is the real-life worst that could happen if these difficult, tough, or hard circumstances or conditions continue, or get worse?
- Could reporting the problem lead to a job loss? How do I handle it or am I prepared for such a consequence?
- At what point do I say "enough is enough"? Or do I endure or stay regardless of the outcome? If I remain, what are the consequences? Are those consequences better/worse than if I took another action?

Problem Solve

Use your **Career/Work/Business Journal** to help you solve problems that come up in your work. For example, you might write down a problem, issue, or decision you are facing, let it rest on the journal page(s) for a few days or week (or a month, if you have that amount of time), and then come back and see if:

- The problem or issue has been resolved or gone away on its own because it was not a serious matter that needed to be attended to or it was a temporary situation
- Someone else who had the necessary resources and authority has resolved the problem

- You have found just the right solution for the situation and were able to implement it and resolve the situation

Why would you want to write down a problem you are facing at work or in business and then come back to it later? For several reasons:

1) It frees and relaxes your mind from having to remember the problem because it has already been captured on the page
2) You have identified several ways to handle it and now only have to decide which one is the best
3) It gives you time away from the problem to not only focus your energies elsewhere but also to destress a bit while letting your subconscious mind percolate or mull over the best solution

It is also a good idea to make a note of the solution that was found to a problem. That way, you can look back in your journal to see how you have handled previous scenarios and be confident that you can solve current and future issues that come up or avoid options which did not work. It would also be beneficial to note the reasons why they did not work as the situation, people, or other conditions may be different in a similar future situation.

Transition to a Career in Health
Do you want to make the transition to a job or career in health, wellness, or medicine? If yes, I would recommend journaling about this from an education and career viewpoint while also considering any effects it could have on your health. That means that you write about the training, courses, practicum, exams, etc. you need to do as part of learning, the financing of your education, and then the work of starting a new career in addition to other aspects of such a change including finding clients, choosing a location to work at, etc.

From a health viewpoint, if you are making a change to a career as a yoga instructor, massage therapist, homeopath or naturopath, nurse, chiropractor, doctor, or another health or wellness path, note how it affects your own health and well-being. Are you getting less sleep because of classes and study time? Or, are you taking better care of yourself by doing more yoga postures on a regular basis, applying knowledge about herbs, or practicing meditation regularly? Tuning into these areas will help you to stay on top of your own health throughout this time.

Notice Your Career's Impact on Your Health
Whether you have been working at your current job for a while or are transitioning to a new career or field of work, it is important to notice the impact that your career has on your health. How is your career affecting your physical, emotional, and mental health? Are you staying active or are you so stressed out by work that you do not have the energy to be active? Are you able to sleep at night or is work keeping you up and awake when you should be sleeping? Do you notice any symptoms showing up recently because there is increased pressure at work?

It is important to be aware and make a note of the impact your job or work has on your health. It is also vital to know whether the stress and impact on your health are short-term or long-term. This can assist you to make a plan and know whether you should implement stress-management techniques to see you through the short-term pressure or begin actively searching for a less stressful job or field to work in or just a different employer.

Prepare for Retirement
Use your journal as a support to prepare yourself for retirement.

Retirement may come when you have planned for it or it may come at a different, and earlier, time than expected due to a layoff, health issue, or another unexpected event. Having a plan for what you want to do in retirement – hobbies, volunteering, starting a new career, spending more time with grandchildren and family – and how you will schedule your day can make for a smoother and easier transition, not just for yourself but also for your spouse and family. You will be prepared for how your days will be structured and you will have a purpose.

You can and should begin planning for this next stage of your life about five years ahead. As an example, if you want to have a new part-time business in retirement, start now with steps to take each year so that you can seamlessly transition to it when the time comes. For instance, if you wish to have a woodworking business, begin to look at training courses and options and the availability of a fully equipped woodworking workshop, whether at home in a part of the garage or at a facility outside of the home. You will want to know ahead of time what steps you need to take to prepare a workshop – build an addition to your home, winterize a garage or workshop, or rent space – and the finances you will need to complete these or other needed steps.

Your journaling time might also include how you feel about retirement and this may bring up a variety of feelings and emotions. Retirement is a new stage of life, so strong feelings and emotions during this period are to be expected to deal with the loss of colleagues, the end of meaningful, enjoyable or well-paid work, or a change in the structure of the day. Journaling may also reveal that, during the working years, some aspects of one's life were left undeveloped or were ignored such as the relationship with one's spouse, participation in civic events, volunteering, helping at church, hobbies, and others.

Journal Through Tough Times
While it is not pleasant to be going through tough or challenging situations, they may present opportunities to grow or change your career or business. For example, by navigating through a tough time or challenging experience, you might discover a need or niche for a product or service that you can then develop, market, and offer. Keep in mind that the possibility of a new business or career, product, or service may not be part of every difficult time or experience. However, it is still something that you can look for or learn from, providing hope and possibilities for the future.

To help you learn more about yourself and discern the situation you are in, below are some questions to ask and answer in your journal:

- What is bringing about or causing these tough times?
- How do the tough or challenging times make me feel?
- Why do I really feel or react that way? Is there some deeper cause or reason than an obvious, visible, or external problem?

What can I do to deal with tough times? What is the most pressing problem?

- Problem: Lack of social contact
  Solution: Ways to handle or prepare for ways to stay in contact with others
- Problem: Lack of job opportunities
  Solution: Plan for and start your own business, attend a career fair, make an appointment at a job resource centre, update your resume, apply for a job, access resources at the library, etc.
- Problem: Inadequate immunity
  Solution: Increase fitness, improve diet, reduce weight, etc.

CAREER/WORK/BUSINESS JOURNAL

It is an exciting opportunity to use your **Career Journal** as a key tool and companion on your journey to realizing your full potential and using your gifts in the work you do! As you take note of your skills and gifts, tasks you like, and hours and locations where you want to work and implement those where you can, you will feel an increased satisfaction and fulfillment in your work as well as take pride in a job well done.

The ways to use your **Career/Work/Business Journal** include to:

- Prepare for Interviews
- Consider Working from Home (see chapter **30. Books – Working from Home**)
- Explore the Option of Hiring a Career or Business Coach
- Give Drawing a Try
- Discover Your Gifts and Talents
- Capture Entrepreneurial Ideas (see chapter **30. Books – Entrepreneurial Ideas**)
- Consider Technology
- Notice If You Are Blazing Your Own Trail or Following In Someone Else's Footsteps
- Identify Negative or Toxic Work Environments
- Problem Solve
- Transition to a Career in Health
- Notice Your Career's Impact on Your Health
- Prepare for Retirement (see chapter **30. Books – Retirement/Second Career**)
- Journal Through Tough Times

Notes

Career/Work/Business Journal

1. Garnet, Barbori. 2021. *Home at the Office: Working Remotely as a Way of Life.* Atmosphere Press.

11

Creativity Journal

"Creativity flourishes when we have a sense of safety and self-acceptance."
"No matter what your age or your life path, whether making art is your career or your hobby or your dream, it is not too late or too egotistical or too selfish or too silly to work on your creativity."
– Julia Cameron, *The Artist's Way*
"…Creativity is God's gift to us. Using creativity is our gift back to God."
– Julia Cameron, *Heart Steps*

It is important to realize that for some, creativity may come in bursts or that it ebbs and flows throughout the days, weeks, and months and that is okay while for others, daily creative expression is a must. When you have ideas and creative insights, make sure to jot those down and capture them as soon as possible (even if it means turning on a flashlight or lamp in the middle of the night; it is also a good idea to keep a notepad next to your bed for this purpose) – you do not want to forget those brilliant moments of creative inspiration!

Creative Ways

The first media that may come to mind for what is considered creative might be art (painting, drawing, sculpture), photography, and writing (short stories, poems, plays, fiction, etc.). In addition to these, consider the following ways of being creative:

1. Drawing
   - pencil
   - pen and ink
   - pastel
   - charcoal
2. Painting
   - watercolor
   - oil
   - acrylic
   - gouache
3. Sculpting
4. Photography
5. Writing
   - poetry
   - short stories
   - fiction
   - non-fiction
   - script writing
   - essays
   - articles
6. Calligraphy
7. Journaling/Art Journaling
8. Bookbinding
9. Scrapbooking
10. Card making

11. Candle making
12. Soap making
13. Composing music
14. Playing an instrument
15. Singing
16. Acting
17. Dancing
18. Filmmaking
19. Jewellery design and making
20. Fashion design
21. Knitting
22. Sewing
23. Crocheting
24. Quilting
25. Baking
26. Cooking
27. Cake decorating
28. Marketing
29. Website coding
30. Website design
31. Problem-solving
32. Organizing your schedule or space
33. Interior Design/Decorating
34. Home staging
35. Floor plan design
36. Furniture design
37. Storage design
38. Gardening
39. Wood carving
40. Woodworking

Keep in mind that there are other ways to be creative, besides those associated with arts, as I share in *Home at the Office: Working Remotely as a Way of Life*: "For example, creativity – was there a time when you offered to help create clever storage solutions for a small space or you saw a problem and already knew how to solve it? Or if you really wanted to do something, were there examples where you rearranged your schedule to be able to participate? You do not need to be creative in the way an artist is creative, but you need to have enough of that gift [of creativity and resourcefulness] to find solutions to problems."

Designing and Decorating
Do you enjoy designing and decorating spaces? Use your creativity journal to draw floor plans, work out color palettes for painting walls in the rooms of your home, or determine decorative pieces for rooms such as carpets, bedding, throw pillows, and more. Move a couch or armchair from one side of the room to the other. Take down one artwork and replace it with another. Replace the floor rug with another one that has a different color/pattern or is a different size. You can journal about how these changes make a difference in how you feel or how you view or think about the area in your home where you made these changes. Those might seem like small ways to be creative but they are important as those are ways to express your creativity and style, and give you permission to acknowledge that you are creative and can be creative.

As you focus on designing and decorating, take some moments to consider how you have designed and decorated the area where you work on a creative goal. For example, if your creative goal is to sew a dress, make a movie or jewelry, do woodworking projects, or draw or paint portraits, is the space efficient and functional as well as versatile, allowing for different stations to work on projects in progress and support you reaching your goal? If you want to sew an outfit, you might have one large desk where you keep fabrics and a sewing machine while on a smaller desk you might place books that are relevant to the task at hand like sewing patterns and techniques or history of sewing and fashion. If you want to draw or paint portraits, you might organize your space by placing a small bust on the corner of a desk while in another area you have an easel setup. Keep in mind, too, that the items you use to decorate your space may have one or more purposes such as decorative (an item that looks nice), practical (reference materials), and motivational (encouraging hard work to reach a goal).

Style and Fashion
What are your favorite accessories – scarves, hats, etc.? Who are your style icons? What jewelry do you prefer to wear – bracelets, necklaces, earrings, rings, or a combination of some or all? What are your favorite clothes and go-to ensembles for different seasons, weather, and occasions? Make a list of articles of clothing or accessories that you may want to find and get in order to improve your current wardrobe. Include pictures – you could even start a vision board for fashion and style – and note videos of styles that you like or do a quick sketch or list of what you see someone dressed in that you would like to wear. There is a lot you can capture and enjoy about style and fashion so have fun with keeping this journal.

Maybe you want to learn about how clothes are made and where fabrics are sourced. A great place to start with this could be choosing one or two of your favorite designers and then doing research into their processes of designing and making clothes. Make a list of questions you have and find those answers. Add to your list as questions come up.

Note your favorite colors of clothes and whether you like a nautical style of clothes, favor classic looks instead, or prefer some other styles. Draw your fashion designs, write down the names of designers and labels you come across that you like, and take note of what shoes you like – all of this and more can be part of your journal. Liking your wardrobe and what you wear can increase your self-confidence and appeal to current or prospective friends, partners, clients, employers, etc.

New Creative Ventures
Do you want to try new creative ventures? Look into community classes or courses/workshops offered by arts centres, art galleries, local libraries, colleges, and other organizations. Make a list of the classes and workshops you would like to take – perhaps theatre or singing or a pottery class – and carve out time in your calendar, set aside the funds in your budget, and then register for the event. Or, as you read articles and stories of how others are being creative, write down the things that resonate with you and that you want to try.

Set Aside Time
Schedule time for being creative. When it is scheduled in your calendar, you will have that time blocked off to dedicate to a creative pursuit or activity. It can be a commitment to a weekly class or maybe you would prefer to set aside one weekend a month to focus entirely on creativity. If you decide to set aside one weekend a month for creative pursuits, what can you do during a dedicated creative time? Below are some practical suggestions, steps, and actions you can take:

- Read books on:
  - Creativity:
  Start More Than You Can Finish by Becky Blades

Writing for Life by Julia Cameron
The Artist's Way by Julia Cameron
The Creative Life by Julia Cameron
Keep Going by Austin Kleon
- Idea Generation:
100 Side Hustles by Chris Guillebeau
- Starting and Running a Successful Business:
Creative, Inc. by Meg Mateo Ilasco and Joy Deangdeelert Cho
- Think of what you like to do. Find out what the choices are for classes and workshops to take, talks to attend, and more. You might discover that there are not many available options to choose from or the offerings are not high quality. If so, list ideas to solve this situation such as:
  - How you would improve it
  - Determine if it could be a viable business by figuring out profit and conditions needed such as space requirements and number of customers
  - What you wish someone would create – a service, a way to do something, or a gadget or tool to use
- Research writing contests to enter, art shows to be part of, residencies to apply for, etc.
- Take inventory of the progress you have made and things you have learned in your creative pursuits and then write down new goals to work toward and accomplish

Another suggestion is to spend 10, 15, or up to 30 minutes a day doing something creative as a way to change up your day from work tasks and family responsibilities.

The amount of time you set aside for being creative may ebb and flow from week to week or month to month. Take notice of it and try to include some set times for creativity as much as you can in order to be consistent and gain confidence in your creative expression. To help you stay on track, make a list of practical actions and steps to achieve your goals and a date by which to achieve them.

Hobby or Career
Another aspect to consider in your journal is whether creativity is a hobby or career either at this stage or time in your life or if, for example, in the future – such as with a move to a different city, province/state or country, in retirement, as children are growing up – you plan to pursue art as a part- or full-time job. Knowing how you view creativity and what role it has in your life – hobby or career – can help you keep things in perspective and make the best decisions. If you find that as you spend more time on creativity as a hobby, and hone your skills, it gradually becomes a career or turns into a job opportunity, that is okay, just be aware that it could happen. A great way to approach this is to list your current hobbies and skills, potential or future hobbies and skills, and how to try the hobbies out and acquire the skills.

For some, daily creativity – whether that is art, photography, music, dance, or writing – is their career. If that is the case, it can be a nice break to switch things up and do a creative project that is unrelated to what you normally do for work. Maybe you might like to doodle, work on a scrapbook, or sing. Choose an outlet that will be fun, enjoyable, and different from your regular creative work.

Stress Management
Creativity is a wonderful avenue through which to both manage and lower stress. You are able to give expression to what you are going through and how you feel or perhaps completely forget about your stress while being immersed in a creative activity. If you are going

through a particularly stressful time, it may be a good idea to set aside more time to be creative to help manage what you are feeling.

If trying a creative pursuit is new for you, it is a good idea to journal how you feel after participating in the creative endeavor. Ask yourself whether or not you feel more relaxed and if you feel a decrease in stress. If not, some things to consider are whether you are feeling internal pressure – your expectations – or external pressure – from family, friends, or others – and why as you do a creative activity. You may want to try a different approach or try another creative outlet entirely to see if it might be a better fit.

Creativity Sharing
As well, think about and consider ways in which you can use your creative gifts to share with and bless others. It is nice to bring a touch of happiness and a smile to the lives of other people through our gifts and talents. Perhaps you can paint or draw a scene on a homemade birthday card for a family member or friend, lead or teach a class or workshop to share your skills and experience, or give suggestions or help decorate a venue for an event. Be prepared that there either can or will be resistance or even push back to your efforts at wanting to share your creative gifts with others.

Writing down your creative goals, the means and timeline or deadline to achieve them, and seeing yourself take steps to achieve them can be an encouragement to you to try new things and grow your skills. Remember, too, that your art and creativity skills are a gift and there are many ways to develop and use those skills and talents.

Your **Creativity Journal** can include these areas to journal about:

- Creative Ways
- Designing and Decorating
- Style and Fashion
- New Creative Ventures
- Setting Aside Time
- Hobby or Career
- Stress Management
- Creativity Sharing

12

Dream Journal

"Dreams are the touchstones of our character."
"If you have built castles in the air, your work need not be lost; that is where they should be. Now put the foundations under them."
– Henry David Thoreau

Before skipping over this chapter thinking it is not for you, give it a chance. You might learn a thing or two about dreams and the importance of vision that can be applied to your journaling.

When Do You Dream?
Record your dreams to discover if you notice any patterns in what you dream about and when you dream most (i.e., is it in the morning before you wake up?). If you have scary or frightening dreams, is it because you watched a scary movie or show before bed? Or watched the news or read a scary book before falling asleep?

Sometimes, our sleep, and therefore our dreams, can be affected by what we eat and how close we eat to bedtime. Take note of the foods you eat before bed and begin to notice which foods encourage or help with better sleep and sweeter dreams.

Dreams from Childhood, Dreams from Now
For most, some dreams change over time from the ones in childhood to those in adulthood. Take some time to write in your journal about your childhood dreams and the dreams you have now. Are they similar or different? In what way(s) are they similar or different and how or why have they changed? Have some of your dreams come true? What dreams did you have of your future when you were young and have some of those come true?

When Dreams Die
Many people think of dreams as an exciting time of new possibilities and ideas to ponder and then put into action step-by-step. While that is one part or side of dreams, the other side is dreams which go unrealized. And that can hurt, be painful, and be uncomfortable, especially if those dreams were near and dear to one's heart. It is okay to acknowledge this other side, or downside, of dreams. If those dreams – the ones near and dear to your heart – were unfulfilled, another way to see this is to ask and answer in your journal what other opportunities you took advantage of instead.

Dreams may die, either because they are no longer ones that a person wants to pursue or because the opportunity for them has passed. When it is the latter, it can be a time of sadness and loss and slowly processing the closing of one opportunity while not yet knowing or being sure of what lies ahead or is opening in the future. If that is what you are experiencing or feeling, know that your journal is the space to explore that and write down what you are going through.

Turning Dreams into Goals
A dream can be the beginning of a goal. In order to turn a dream into reality, a plan of action – a series of goals – must be put into place. During your journaling time, write down the dreams that come to mind and then take the time to think about, pray, and seek guidance to know which one(s) to turn into goals and work on achieving.

As you become reacquainted with yourself, you will begin to fill your journal with and discover dreams tucked away from many years ago as well as more recently formed hopes and dreams. Enjoy this time of uncovering what you hold important and cherish in your life. A **Dream Journal** can be used as a tool to learn more about what you envision for your future. Here are some topics to cover in your journal:

- When Do You Dream?
- Dreams from Childhood, Dreams from Now
- When Dreams Die
- Turning Dreams into Goals

13

Education/Learning Journal

"The only thing that is more expensive than education is ignorance."
"An investment in knowledge pays the best interest."
– Benjamin Franklin

The joy of learning and education is that they are a lifelong pursuit. There is no age at which learning stops nor does it end with high school or post-secondary. For some, it will feel as if true, interest-led learning starts once formal education finishes. Continue reading for ideas on how to approach education and learning during your time of journaling.

Lifelong Learning
Write down things you want to learn, facts or interesting information you have come across (such as from watching a *Jeopardy!* episode or reading an e-mail), or quotes about learning and education that you find inspiring. Take your journal with you when you go to a talk or lecture. Have your journal beside you as you listen to a webinar. Jot down anything that stands out to you such as:

- Mentions of links, books, podcasts, or other resources you want to remember and take a look at or listen to later on
- Questions you want to ask the speaker or presenter during Q&A time
- Other topics, facts, or statistics that you want to look into to learn more about or understand better
- Opinions, viewpoints, or ideas you might disagree with and note why you disagree and what would be a better solution along with why and how to implement or achieve a better outcome
- Further talks or presentations you would like to attend to continue your learning journey

Learning should be an ongoing pursuit throughout each person's life. Learning does not end with formal education (high school, post-secondary, etc.) nor is it limited to take place only on professional development days or during continuing education classes.

Just as I have, you can use your journal to list the pros and cons of a program or degree you are considering to help you decide whether or not to pursue it. That being said, however, formal education such as going back to school for a program or degree or taking continuing education classes are only two of the ways in which you can pursue lifelong learning. Other places and ways to gain knowledge from include:

- Accessing resources at the library and attending courses offered there
- Listening to podcasts
- Looking up books and magazines related to the topic you want to learn about and reading relevant chapters and articles
- Being a mentor and/or mentee. As a mentor, you need to refresh,

deepen, and update your knowledge on a regular basis in order to assist or support your mentee in their areas of growth
- Joining an organization of interest to you. Experts and masters pass on their experience and knowledge to you through demonstrations and talks
- Being part of a book club can lead to discussions prompted by:
  - Questions provided at the end of the book
  - Opening a discussion on themes or topics of interest
  - Other members' experiences and insights
- Attending lectures, seminars, workshops, talks, presentations, conferences, etc. Specialists in the field are up-to-date in knowledge and research and can provide comparisons of the past and present, development and progress, what needs or is left to be done now, and useful reference materials.

You can attend a series of weekly classes or go to a two-hour or one-day workshop once a month or once a quarter. You can also learn by going to events in person, watching and listening online, or a combination of the two. As you actively welcome and engage in learning opportunities, be prepared for the variety of topics you will come across and begin learning about.

Homeschooling and Children's Education

Are you homeschooling or thinking of homeschooling your children? If yes, an **Education/Learning Journal** is the perfect place to write down ideas and suggestions for classes and online courses, resources, textbooks, and school boards that you are considering and want to come back to later on to become familiar with. You might also draft an outline or scope of learning for the coming school year for your children.

It may be helpful and encouraging to know that learning does not require a lot of expense or cost. Rather, there are so many options and possibilities for ongoing education that can fit your budget while exploring new topics and subjects and gaining skills and knowledge!

A journal can be a great support along the homeschooling journey. Include ideas for field trips you can take with your children, unit studies to do, and books to read. To encourage you on your homeschooling path, write down:

- Articles and books to read
- Curricula and resources to look into
- Subjects and interests your children enjoy or areas where more attention or time is needed
- The dates and locations of homeschool conventions and conferences you would like to attend
- Anything else that would be helpful to remember or want to refer to at a later time

It is a privilege and blessing to be able to homeschool one's children. It may not be easy and you may encounter or face difficulties and challenges along the way. However, everything worthwhile or worth doing never comes with any guarantee that it will be easy or smooth sailing.

A homeschooling journal could also be an opportunity to introduce your kids to journaling. They could write about:

- What they have learned while taking a field trip, reading a book, or playing outside with siblings or friends
- What they want to learn more about and do research on

- Experiments they want to try
- Games they want to play
- Plays and music performances they want to organize
- Music pieces they want to learn
- Math lessons they want to apply in real life such as starting a business, learning to budget, going grocery shopping, planting a garden, designing and making a woodworking project, etc.

Their journal could include sketches, drawings, maps, clippings, and more. A journal can be a place to let the imagination be free as well as a record of how much your children have learned.

Your Education – What Was It Like?
What were your school years like? How did they affect you? What do you need to unlearn? In what ways do you want your children's education to be different? We might not pick up on or be aware of it but what we learn and the way it was taught can have an effect on us: why we chose a certain major or degree in post-secondary, whether we like to learn independently or not, and how we approach research and studying.

Other areas to think about are whether education was valued in your family as being important for both boys and girls or whether you were encouraged to learn and excel and aspire to achieve by taking courses and attending post-secondary.

Over time, your **Education/Learning Journal** will show you how much you have learned, what you tried, and where you have matured. By embracing ongoing learning, you may discover and develop new interests, hobbies, social groups, and friends.

EDUCATION/LEARNING JOURNAL

Areas and topics to journal about in an **Education/Learning Journal** can include:

- Lifelong Learning
- Homeschooling and Children's Education
- Your Education – What Was It Like?

14

Family History Journal

> "The thing that interests me most about family history is the gap between the things we think we know about our families and the realities."
> – Jeremy Hardy

The stories and histories that are passed down in families are part of what makes us who we are and can influence our future, too. Shared in this chapter are some areas to consider as you explore family history.

Family Letters, Journals, Diaries, or Records
Perhaps you have inherited a collection of letters or diaries from someone in your family or the journals have been handed down from generation to generation. Treasure these volumes for the stories, experiences, teachings and learnings, and wisdom they contain and share.

Depending on the content of historical family letters and journals, it may be appropriate and you may decide (after consulting other family members, if needed) to temporarily loan them to a museum for an exhibit (you might want to look into valuations, insurance, and legal requirements first). Another good idea would be to ensure that your family's letters and journals from previous generations are properly preserved for future generations. If translations or restorations are needed, find knowledgeable professionals who have experience and expertise in these areas.

Family Behaviors and Patterns
Another side of family history is to journal about both positive and negative patterns and behaviors as well as notice what effects – again, both positive and negative – those have had on you and in your relationships and interactions with others: spouse/partner, children, friends, extended family, neighbors, colleagues, and maybe even pets and animals. It may not be easy to think about these instances from your past or family of origin. However, if relationships and interactions are to improve for the better not just now but also for the next generations, the time and effort must be put into this to analyze and correct where needed.

In addition, part of your entries could include what you imagine your ancestors went through – struggles and challenges, joys and celebrations – especially if they immigrated and settled in a new place. You could also delve into how the challenges your ancestors faced shaped their character, attitudes (especially toward money or finances and discipline), and outlook for the future (optimistic vs. pessimistic, security-oriented, ambitious, etc.).

Family Traditions
A **Family History Journal** is the perfect place to capture your family's favorite and special traditions, both those kept alive from generation to generation and newer ones. Did your grandparents have a special

recipe or tradition at Christmas time? Write that down so that you can remember it and share and pass it on to other family members. Did you and your siblings have a favorite song you sang for each other's birthdays or a game you always played during summer vacation while camping or at the family cottage? These are all moments to remember and preserve now to be able to share with the next generations.

Or, maybe your family did not have many traditions. If that is the case, use your journal to jot down ideas for traditions you would like to begin. That way, you can come back to your journal to remember how and when to give the new tradition a try.

Another way to utilize your journal is to make a list of questions to ask family members – such as about their growing up years, traveling abroad, being in the military, relatives' names, occupations, why ancestors moved from one place to another, or if there is a reason why names are spelled differently and different names show in different records – and write down their answers. You could also make a list of family members to record as they tell their life stories so that they would be preserved in audio format.

Enjoy the journey of unearthing more about your family's history and how it relates to the present. Keep your journal close by to record what you find and feelings, thoughts, and memories that may come up during this process.

A **Family History Journal** can incorporate these areas:

- Family Letters, Journals, Diaries, or Records
- Family Behaviors and Patterns
- Family Traditions

15

Gardening/Home Journal

"Flowers always make people better, happier, and more helpful; they are sunshine, food and medicine for the soul."
– Luther Burbank

"Where flowers bloom, so does hope."
– Lady Bird Johnson

Gardening is an activity to take delight in, both as a hands-on gardener and as a viewer who admires the beauty of tenderly cared-for yards one encounters on walks and in parks. Gardening-related journaling can add appreciation for the beauty of and changes in nature from season to season and year to year. Because our homes are where we welcome loved ones, taking the time to stay on top of projects and maintenance in a journal can help keep things manageable.

How Does Your Garden Grow?
Keeping a gardening journal to record how and when your garden grows can be rewarding to keep and look back on. You can include photos of plants, trees, bushes, flowers, vegetables, and fruits in your journal to help you remember the plentiful blossoms, the colors of

plants in your yard, the bountiful harvest, or how your garden has changed over the years (height of trees, new beds, potted plants, etc.). Other information you may like to include in a gardening journal is:

- The names of seeds sown and plants planted
- Step-by-step instructions for how you built a raised bed, cold frame, or other structure
- Newspaper or magazine articles with special or important gardening instructions
- The date you planted seeds, the first sign of seedlings, the first tree or bush to flower, when crocuses or tulips peak through in the spring, the first frost, the first snowfall, and more
- Your plans and ideas for planting and growing an Herb garden, Perennial Flower bed, Bee-Friendly garden, or Vegetable garden

It can be interesting to compare your entries from year to year as you may notice that plants have flowered earlier or later depending on the weather each year. For example, by keeping a gardening journal, I have been able to review previous years and note the different times each spring that an apricot tree in my family's backyard flowered, which has varied by up to a month over a few years.

There are many who have kept journals of their gardens over the years. You might also like to peruse your favorite gardening books and magazines as these can be great sources of inspiration and ideas to you for your own garden. Jot down the book or magazine titles and page numbers of things you find so that you could refer back to it later if needed.

Fragrances
When you walk around your garden or a garden in a park, take time to

breathe in and notice the fragrances of flowers. Some of the ones you might notice, and a few of my favorites, are:

- Lilac bushes
- Mayday trees
- Mock orange bushes
- Allysum flowers
- Petunia flowers
- Roses

What does the fragrance remind you of or conjure memories of? For example, it could be that the scent of lilacs reminds you of your mother or grandmother – perhaps lilac was your mother's or grandmother's favorite flower.

Gardening or Horticultural Club
Whether attending your first or fiftieth meeting, bring your journal to gardening or horticultural club meetings. The meetings are a good time to write down the names of plants mentioned, growing tips and techniques, planting suggestions, garden plans, and more. If there are guest speakers at meetings, you can take notes of what advice for care of plants and gardens was shared. You can also make notes of tips you would like to share with the other members. Seeing the collection of notes over time from gardening or horticultural club meetings will show how much knowledge you have gained and learned.

DIY/Project/Home Maintenance
For projects and maintenance around the home, a great way to stay on top of these is to make a list of:

- Things you need or want to make or improve

- Track progress
- Supplies to buy
- Skills to learn
- Tasks to do each day/week/month to make progress

Consider whether you will need to hire a professional or if you can ask for assistance from friends, family, or neighbors. If someone recommends a plumber, electrician, carpenter, home renovator or builder, architect, landscaper, permaculturist, etc., write down the contact information of the person or company in your journal. You can also write down the steps to do certain projects so that you can save time in doing the project the next time.

Keeping a garden/home journal over the years can be rewarding. It provides a place to go back and review not only how much you have grown and learned as a gardener but also the ways in which your yard has changed and grown. Use your **Gardening/Home Journal** for the following:

- Noticing How Your Garden Grows
- Fragrances
- Gardening or Horticultural Club
- DIY/Project/Home Maintenance

16

Goals Journal

"Everyone needs a concrete, specific goal — an ambition, and a purpose — to limit chaos and make intelligible sense of his or her life."
– Jordan Peterson

A **Goals Journal** can be filled with all of the goals you have in many different areas of life: career or job, travel, projects, and others.

Timeline of Goals
Keep in mind that goals can be short-term (up to 2 years), mid-term (2 to 5 years), and long-term (5 or more years) in length and you can include goals from each of these time ranges or just focus on one of these in your journal. In addition to those, consider these timelines of goals that give a specific timeframe:

- New Year's goals: These are usually started at the commencement of a new calendar year, January 1. New Year's goals can be a combination of goals for the year – such as a place to travel to or number of books to read – as well as monthly goals.
- Daily, Weekly, and Monthly Goals: Goals can be pared down into

short-term (daily or weekly goals or tasks) while still helping to work toward mid- or long-term goals (monthly or yearly goals)
- <u>Seasonal Goals:</u> Winter, spring, summer, and fall, new goals can be set or time can be taken to review goals and progress at the beginning of or in each season
- <u>Quarterly Goals:</u> This can align with the seasons or be set for the quarterly period that works best for you

You may decide to have a separate journal for each goal that you have, to keep to-do items and completed steps separate and organized, or write about all your goals in one notebook. Or, you might prefer to keep track of short-term goals and mid- or long-term goals in separate journals to ensure everything is streamlined.

Time

In addition to addressing the length of time it might take to reach your goals, it is important to use your journal to help you discover if you are spending enough time on your goals. If your goal is to write and publish a novel in the next two years, are you blocking enough time in your calendar today, this week, and this month to make that a reality? If extra projects at work or responsibilities at home will increase or decrease, what changes can you make to your schedule to have the time to make some progress on your goals? Utilize your journal to assist you in identifying how you are currently using your time and where you could make adjustments.

Energy

How much of your energy is being put toward actually and actively working on your goals compared to avoiding or delaying working on them? If this is the case, ask yourself in your journal why this is happening. Is it because the goal that has been set is not right for you or not right at this time but maybe in three or six months might be a better timing? Has the goal been properly formulated – is it measurable? Vagueness may siphon off energy before you even begin by being unsure or indecisive. Do you have resources to expend the energy on the effort? Do you have the needed support? Try rewording or redirecting your goals by looking for the reasons for this situation.

Knowing how your energy is being directed in the area of your goals is vital to understanding what is going on and being able to find solutions. Are you feeling discouraged or is the focus of your goal in some way emotionally, mentally, or physically demanding? Most goals, besides requiring time and planning, require some form of energy such as:

- The energy of critical thinking, careful thought, and the need for personal, quiet time to recharge
- The energy of physical activity or exertion
- The energy of emotional investment
- The energy of self-confidence and going in the right direction

Which one – or more – of the above do each one of your goals demand of you? Being aware of what energy you will need to give to your projects will also help you prepare for ways to replenish your energy and schedule time to recharge.

Learning and Growing
A benefit of setting and working toward goals is the opportunity to learn or develop further – specific skills, perseverance, planning, and organization – and then to grow from that experience and apply the lessons learned to future plans or situations.

Another way to view learning and growing in relation to goals is to know who and when to ask for advice. Potential people to turn to when advice is needed are a parent, sibling, other family member, friend, or mentor. Wisdom and discernment are required to determine who to turn to and be able to trust with receiving advice that is for your best.

Supporting Others
Another view to consider is whether you take an active role in supporting others to reach their goals and visions for the future or if you have sabotaged or derailed their goals. Some things to consider are:

- Do you speak words of encouragement and support to cheer others on in reaching their goals and visions for the future?
- Or do you create obstacles or drag your feet, draining the energy of others who are trying to achieve their goals? Draining the energy of others may also hinder you from focusing on your goals.
- Do you share resources – book recommendations, website links or YouTube videos, contest or job opportunities – to help others find and access the tools they need to reach their goals?
- Are you showing up by attending important events, freeing up time by taking care of to-do items, and assisting in creating a dedicated work or studio space for others to reach their goals? In the case of family members, assisting to make a dedicated work or studio space would mean that supplies and projects could be kept in one place rather than in several locations throughout the house, thus helping with overall organization as well as use and enjoyment of the home by all family members.

Supporting Yourself
Do your current habits help, hinder, or block your goals? Giving this some thought could be critical to the future success or failure of your

goals and vision. Do you reflect on or pray for wisdom and guidance as you make decisions regarding your goals? Do you seek wise counsel from others? Do you wake up and go to bed on time in order to have sufficient time and energy to complete the things you need to do to turn your goals into reality? Asking yourself these questions will go a long way in determining whether or not, and how, you are supporting or sabotaging yourself in reaching your vision for the future.

Vision Board
Sometimes, having a board with a collection of images that represent your vision and goals can make it clearer to see and know what you are working toward and want to achieve. Find photos and images that look like your vision for the future and arrange them – on a board, on poster paper, or another material of your choice – in a way that is inspiring to you and provides encouragement.

Planning ahead for and working toward goals are times of excitement and filled with activity to reach the destination. In keeping a **Goals Journal**, these are areas you can focus on to help you stay on track:

- Timeline of Goals
- Time
- Energy
- Learning and Growing
- Supporting Others
- Supporting Yourself
- Vision Board

17

Gratitude Journal

"Piglet noticed that even though he had a Very Small Heart, it could hold a rather large amount of Gratitude."
– A. A. Milne

Life is a gift and a blessing and there is much to be thankful for. By starting and keeping a **Gratitude Journal**, you have a tool in your hand that is an antidote to feelings of depression and anxiety as well as a friend during tough times. Keep this journal close by so that you can write down things you are grateful for as they come up throughout the day.

What Are You Thankful For?
Are you thankful for good health, healing, fresh food, loving and supportive family and friends, safe travels, comfortable living quarters, an inspiring studio, or any number of other things you are blessed with and enjoy? Make it a habit to write in your journal about the people, places, work, and things you are thankful for. Some days, more items may go forth from the pen onto the journal page and that is okay. On the days when it is harder to write about what you are thankful for,

look back at previous entries to remind yourself that you are provided for and what you enjoy.

Write Thank Yous
A journal is a very good place to draft and write thank-you letters. If there is someone you want to thank, but never got the chance to because they have since passed away or you understand now the reason why something was said or done, you can write a thank you to whomever you need to in the space of your journal.

The thank-you letters or notes written in a journal can help to express feelings, emotions, and associations. After writing a thank you, you can decide whether or not it needs to be given or sent.

Take the opportunity to write thank-you notes as you feel prompted. You may discover that you recall a smile, an act of kindness, or a thoughtful gift that made your day or was just the encouragement you needed to make it through a difficult period or challenging time.

A Topic a Day
Each day, you can choose from the below list a different area of your life or topic to express gratitude for:

- The gift of life
- Work and the enjoyment and satisfaction of a job well done
- Good quality items made with skill and craft
- God's love, grace, and plan for redemption
- Love from and for family and friends
- Health and wellness
- The beauty of nature: mountains, beaches, water, forests and their sounds, jungles and their mysteries, deserts, the four seasons each

year, flowers, harvest, the weather
- A warm, comfortable place to call home, rest in, and sleep in
- Skills, talents, and abilities
- Dreams, hopes, goals, and plans
- Places to explore and things to try and do
- Fresh, flavorful food that provides nourishment, energy, and health

Whichever area you choose to focus on, remove the pressure from yourself of feeling that you need to write extensively, for example, writing at least one page. Instead, be genuine in your expression of gratitude even if that means writing one sentence or a short paragraph.

Taking a Break
What if you are not having the best day and do not feel like writing what you are grateful for? That is okay. You do not have to do a gratitude journal entry every day. Instead, you could simply read through what you have written on previous days. Or, you could skip journaling altogether for that day.

The benefits of journaling on a regular basis include having consistent times of slowing down and reflecting on feelings and happenings, conveying gratitude, and knowing what your priorities and goals are to determine if you are applying your energy where needed. While it is best to journal on a regular basis, it is up to you to decide when and how often to journal. You can also choose whether you want to journal during low moments and days or wait until you are feeling a bit more grounded before jotting down thoughts, feelings, emotions, experiences, and more.

Keeping a gratitude journal can help you have a more balanced perspective on life. While this may be a cliché, a **Gratitude Journal** can remind you of the many blessings you have received as well as minimize negative thoughts. These areas can help you with keeping this kind of journal:

- Noting What You Are Thankful For
- Writing Thank Yous
- Selecting a Topic a Day
- Taking a Break

18

Health Journal

"I believe that the greatest gift you can give your family and the world is a healthy you."
– Joyce Meyer

"Writing is medicine. It is an appropriate antidote to injury. It is an appropriate companion for any difficult change."
– Julia Cameron, *The Right to Write*

A **Health Journal** can be a very informative and important key in your journey to reaching and maintaining your health goals. Here are a few different ways to make the most of your journal to support you along your health journey.

Diet, Food, and Recipes
Tracking your diet, the foods you eat and like and do not like, and recipes to make can help you know what foods to buy and meals to prepare. Make note of foods and meals you enjoy as well as meals and recipes you want to learn to make. This type of journal could also incorporate meal tracking and calorie counting.

You can record recipes you have received from others and write down favorite recipes you have made yourself and want to remember. This type of journal can be a great way to help you learn to cook or improve your culinary skills in this area while at the same time honing your recipe selection skills and creating a recipe collection.

Exercise and Fitness
Keep on top of your exercise and fitness goals. Information to include could be:

- Body measurements and weight
- Number of daily steps
- The type of exercises done along with the number of sets and reps
- A weekly or monthly exercise plan to see regular progress in achieving weight loss goals or be able to run a half or full marathon

By noting your goals and seeing the steps you are taking to achieve them, you will be inspired by the progress you make on the journey to improve your health.

Commit to Your Health
Make a commitment to do regular things that are good for your health. Examples of this would be to:

- Jump on a rebounder trampoline for a few minutes on a daily basis
- Get outside for a thirty-minute walk five times a week and record how much sun or daily light exposure you get
- Drink eight glasses of water every day
- Work with a health coach on a weekly or monthly basis
- Make fresh juices and wheatgrass juice two to three times a week
- Commit to one massage a month

Committing to and taking action to maintain your health will help you feel and be your best both in the short term and long term.

Restorative Journaling Techniques
Another aspect of journaling, whether for health and wellness or as part of keeping a health journal to track habits and more, is to ensure that your writing and journaling time is restorative. Here are some suggestions:

- Sit in a position or on something that helps you feel restored: half or full lotus, couch, chair, armchair, hammock, grass, or sand, supported with pillows or blankets
- Only write for as long as it feels good and you have the energy for. If you have more to say but you feel tired, simply capture in point form or in the margins the topics you want to journal about next time
- Start and finish your journaling time by taking deep breaths

Names and Referrals
Write down the names of doctors and other medical and health professionals that friends, family, and neighbors recommend. Writing this down in one place - your journal - means that the information will be easy to access. Jot down notes and follow-up questions on prescriptions given to you by doctors, research into supplements, and anything else necessary to record that relates to your health and well-being.

Include health-related web addresses to visit and books to read in the future. List the names of herbs, adaptogens, and vitamins you want to learn more about that you think would support your health.

Remember, when it comes to your health, you are your own best advocate and your journal is the perfect place to record important information.

Ask Questions

If, for example, you are wanting to increase the quality or length of your sleep, there are several ways that your health journal can help you discover your current patterns before bed to determine what is and is not working:

- What foods are you eating before bed and how close before bed do you finish eating? How does the eating pattern affect your sleep?
- Is there an herbal tea you make and sip before bed which you have noticed has helped you fall asleep sooner or helped you stay asleep?
- Did your sleep improve after going to a relaxing exercise class, such as Yin Yoga, before bed?
- Does it help to have a ritual before going to bed, such as listening to relaxing music, having a cup of tea, reviewing your day or planning for the next day and preparing to-do items, meditating, or doing guided imagery?

You may also want to track how much sleep you get and if other factors, such as daily sun exposure, etc., affect the quality and length of your sleep.

Other health-related areas that you may want to address in your journal to track over time and provide insight into are:

- Exercises and workouts that help you lose weight, get toned, and have more energy
- Exercise/sport/fitness (yoga, Pilates, HIIT, etc.) classes that you

want to try
- For women – note things about your menstrual cycles and hormones
- Specific teas or recipes or other tools you want to try to assist you in achieving optimal health and energy levels
- How your work or job(s) affects your health (increased stress or anxiety, sitting for long periods of time, eating to deal with stress, etc.) and any steps you can take to make positive changes to how you feel
- Activities, meetings, events, or people that leave you feeling either energized or drained of your energy
- Events, people, or weather that trigger a tension headache
- How you feel after a massage. You can try different kinds of massage, as some might leave you feeling more energized while others might make you feel more relaxed
- Questions you have for a doctor or other medical professional to ask during your next appointment
- Discover resources that are available for you to learn more about your diagnosis/condition:
  - Books
  - DVDs/movies
  - Podcasts
  - Workshops
  - Websites
  - Webinars
  - Seminars
  - Audio/CDs
  - Health summits
- Find a library you can go to – at a hospital or other clinic – that has books, DVDs/movies, and more that you can take a look at
- Note treatments or prescriptions that are being strongly recom-

mended or suggested as "the standard of care" but which you do not feel comfortable about following

The above is only a beginning of the questions you can ask yourself and journal your thoughts and feelings about.

Where Do You Carry Stress?
When it comes to stress in your life, be aware and pay attention to where tension shows up in your body. Do you carry it in your shoulders and neck or in your hips? Do you develop nervous tics or twitching? Does your stomach get butterflies or feel queasy, or does your jaw become tense or do you grind your teeth when you are nervous, overwhelmed, or stressed? Do you have heart palpitations or do you hyperventilate? These are just some indications of stress in the body, but each person is different and stress may demonstrate itself in many other bodily reactions.

As you become aware of where you carry stress, use your journal to find ways to bring attention to those areas. Some suggestions include taking deep breaths, doing some stretches, or wearing a mouth guard or retainer to prevent damage to your teeth by grinding. Pay attention to these early signs to prevent major health challenges later on.

Career's Effect on Health
Take note of the effect your career has on your health. As mentioned above, try to notice how your body reacts when a stressful situation or event arises, in this case at work. Do you get butterflies in your stomach or does your heart begin to race? In work, deadlines change, a request is made at the last minute, a key document for an important presentation is misplaced before the presentation time, someone on the team is not being friendly or is withholding information – be aware

of how you react to different situations to know the effect it has on your health and then journal to determine your next course of action.

Keeping a **Health Journal** can help in all of the below areas of setting health goals and staying on track to reach those goals:

- Diet, Food, and Recipes
- Exercise and Fitness
- Commit to Your Health
- Restorative Journaling Techniques
- Names and Referrals
- Ask Questions
- Where You Carry Stress
- Career's Effect on Health

19

Interests Journal

"Interest is the most important thing in life; happiness is temporary, but interest is continuous."
– Georgia O'Keeffe

Book Journals, Movie Journals, Hiking Journals – all these journal subjects and more are great for capturing your interests! Interests and hobbies add a pleasant variety to life.

Books, Music, Art, and Ideas Gained From Reading
I like to write down the titles and authors of books I have enjoyed reading or learned something from. That way, I can look back and not only be reminded of what I have learned and read (and can reference later) but also how much richer my life is for having read so many interesting and varied books and stories. You may prefer writing a book review, along with the book details such as the title and author, to help you remember the main and important ideas shared in the pages.

Through recording details about the books as well as the movies, TV series, songs, music, and art that you like, you will notice that you begin to develop your own list of favorites. By putting together your own collection of top selections, you may also notice that certain themes, topics, and subjects run through the books, movies, etc. that you like - make note of what you like or do not like, feelings that come up, and what the reasons are for your partiality. Then, continue this list of your top choices so that the titles on the list can become the start of your own home library or movie collection, art gallery, or personal playlist and add to those as you find similar titles that you like.

Whether reading fiction or nonfiction books or listening to audiobooks, I encourage you to take the time to slow down and ponder the information you are reading. Engage with the viewpoints presented in the books by writing down what you learn and discover, characters, situations, thoughts, plots, views or ideas that you agree or disagree with and why, and what you connect with, want to emulate or want to avoid. Use this as a means to help you discover other books that you will like, recognize things in your life to work on, and explore ideas you want to examine or put into action.

Movies
Just like journaling ideas from books, the same can be done for journaling about movies you have watched. Perhaps you want to note who directed a movie or who designed the costumes - as an example, I have begun noticing the movies that Edith Head designed costumes for. Or, you might like to write down memorable quotes made by the characters or make a list of movie locations to visit while traveling or on holiday.

Books, Movies, and Their Characters
In books and movies, what do you admire in a character and want to develop in yourself? Qualities you might notice in a character include:

- Loyalty
- Honesty
- Faithfulness
- Leadership
- Kindness
- Sense of adventure
- Unconditional love
- Resourcefulness
- Grace
- Courage
- Perseverance
- Unwavering support
- Creativity
- Integrity
- Generosity

Write down the characters' specific actions or words spoken that show the above qualities. You can also jot down ideas for how you would act or speak in similar situations as the characters find themselves in. You could also write what you would avoid doing or handle differently from the way characters have handled situations in the book's or movie's story.

Hiking and Camping
Keeping a journal on the hiking and camping adventures you have gone on is a great way to remember your time outdoors. Jot down where you encountered breathtaking viewpoints, interesting terrain, wildlife sightings, and favorite campsites that you especially liked because of the level ground for setting up a tent, the right mix of sun and shade, a spacious site, or some other features that you noticed.

This type of journal, or section of an **Interests Journal**, can help you stay organized and remember key information such as writing down when reservations open for campsites, the driving distance - hours or kilometers/miles - to favorite or new hikes or campgrounds, and how long a hike took or notes on elevation gain. You can also keep a list of gear and equipment to take on camping and hiking trips to ensure efficient packing and minimize packing time.

Learning a Language
What is your reason for learning a new language? Is it to converse with a family member, perhaps a grandparent, or a friend? Or do you need to learn a language for your career or to satisfy a graduation or school requirement? Write in your journal your reason for learning a language as this can provide the motivation and encouragement needed to keep making progress.

Learning a new language can open opportunities for conversations with others, enjoy different cultural experiences in your area, or provide a chance to travel to other countries. Along the journey of learning a new language, use your journal as a place to recognize roots to English words, practice writing the alphabet of a language, note pronunciations, and list books, audio, videos, websites and other resources to support your learning adventure. In addition, you can try journaling in a new language to practice and become familiar with structuring sentences, writing, and thinking in the language.

Helping Prepare for Retirement
Another excellent way to utilize an **Interests Journal** would be to help you prepare for retirement. How would you approach this in your journal? About five years in advance of retirement, write down all the things that you enjoy and could do to fill your time. It is vital to

your mental, physical, and emotional health – and that of your family members – to keep active and remain interested and engaged in life throughout your retirement years. Examples and suggestions for what to do to stay active in retirement include:

- Volunteering at a thrift store, animal shelter, language class, the library, car repair or woodworking workshops (these positions enable hands-on skills and practical knowledge to be passed on to younger generations), etc.
- Starting a home-based or online business
- Taking continuing education classes or pursuing a diploma or degree
- Starting a new hobby or returning to a hobby from long ago
- Learning to play an instrument, beginning a garden or expanding your current garden space, taking up woodworking, or pursuing another hands-on interest of your choice
- Mentoring, spending time, and sharing your wisdom with younger colleagues or the younger generation in your fields of expertise

What Interests You?
Perhaps you have been focused on work, looking after your family, or completing education for several years. Now, you find you have more time and would like to become reacquainted with yourself again.

Start with this: Ask yourself what your interests are and what you find interesting. Your answers to these will help you determine what your next step is for what you want to learn more about and explore. You may decide to pursue some interests on your own while other interests may be great to do with friends or family. Enjoy this time of discovering new ideas and potential future activities.

An **Interests Journal** is the perfect help to become reacquainted with your interests and what you find interesting, both now and what you would like to pursue in the future. These are some areas to write about in your journal:

- Books, Music, Art, and Ideas Gained From Reading
- Movies
- Books, Movies, and Their Characters
- Hiking and Camping
- Learning a Language
- Helping Prepare for Retirement
- What Interests You

20

Life Journal

"My pen shall heal, not hurt."
– L.M. Montgomery

Taking time to record everyday happenings, even just a half page or full page daily, can help you remember seemingly ordinary things and realize how rich your life is. From a colorful sunrise to a quiet evening with a cup of tea or a stroll through a park, or a lovely lunch with a friend to a new client or business opportunity, our lives are filled with blessings and special moments. Although these things or moments may seem mundane, by writing them down, you will be able to read over and be reminded – through good and difficult times – that you are provided for, that there were and will again be beautiful moments. This gives you a record of activities bringing pleasure, calm, relaxation, or excitement which will tide you over a period of boredom, stress, disappointment, or even grief.

Personal and Family Relationships
For some journalers, it might be a right fit to journal about personal relationships in a **Life Journal**. Remember that it is your journal so

however much or little you choose to write about relationships is up to you. However, writing about things that happened may help you see what you may not have noticed before, such as repeated actions or behavior patterns. Being aware of these insights can then assist you in determining whether there are any changes to make or actions to take.

You can also write about the little (or big) things that you know make family members and/or your partner feel special and loved and the things that others in your family have done for you that have made you feel that you are a priority in their lives. Other great ideas are to write down gift and date ideas as they come up, mention how family reunions, dates with a partner or other family events/partner outings have gone, and list gifts received. Use your journal to help you in any relationships, and process anything that is going on, whether that is with family, friends, or children.

By journaling about relationships or specific areas of relationships, you might realize that there are certain behaviors or reactions that are occurring that need to be addressed. Proceed by understanding what is going on and make adjustments or changes where and as needed. Journaling on a regular basis can be a tool to help you process what you are going through. Your journal can also be a place to write and reflect your way through any decisions you need to make.

Personal Journey
Your journal is the place where you write about your life, your experiences, and your personal journey called life. It is the place you can record:

- Wins
- Losses

- Beginnings
- Endings
- Changes
- Transitions
- Setbacks
- Surprises
- Promotions
- Disappointments
- Goals
- Ideas
- Fears
- Love
- Friendships
- Joys
- Plans
- Hopes

It can also be helpful to keep in mind that your personal journey in life is unique and will be different from the journeys of others. Events such as marriage, education, and starting and finishing jobs and careers will happen at different times from those of your friends, family, neighbors, colleagues, or whoever else may be in your social circle.

Family History
Perhaps you remember the special dishes your mother or grandmother would make at holidays or birthdays. Or, maybe your family went to the cottage every summer and you recall the fun times you had playing with your cousins. Do you remember falling asleep to stories your mom or dad would read to you or tell at bedtime?

Make your journal the special space where you recollect and record the much-loved family traditions, meals, moments, holidays, and more. Writing it down now will help you to remember loved ones and feel connected with your family. You will also have a place where you can go when you want to remind yourself of the memorable times and perhaps also something to share with other family members such as younger generations.

Decisions and Fear
A helpful way to use a journal is to notice how you make decisions. Do you make decisions out of fear and what-ifs of what others might do or what might happen? Or do you make decisions with hope and courage, trusting that each step of the way will become clear at the right time?

You can also look back on decisions you have made in the past to see whether you decided based on fear, courage, or some combination of the two and what the results have been. Then, you can determine what changes, if any, you need to make to your decision-making process in order to begin or continue to make decisions with courage, faith, hope, and trust.

Acting with Courage
Life is full of highs and lows, joys and disappointments. It is okay to journal about all of these ebbs and flows in your life. If you record these moments and happenings, you can look back and see times that are significant in your life. An example of this might be a time where you summoned and showed a great deal of inner strength, for instance, having the courage to do what was right even in the face of adversity or opposition. Being reminded of this can then give you renewed hope and strength to persevere through current challenges or setbacks you may be facing.

Dreams, Hopes, Plans
A **Life Journal** may also include your dreams, hopes, and wishes, as well as plans for the future. Once again, reviewing these may provide just the encouragement you might need when you encounter difficulties. Whatever moments, thoughts, and experiences you decide to journal on and include in your journal, remember that life is a gift and blessing worth celebrating and sharing.

Intuition
Do you listen to your intuition? This requires listening to the still, small voice inside. Over the years, your intuition may have been ignored or shut down in ways that may seem harmless. For example, when you were a child you may have been told to hug someone even if you did not want to because you felt uncomfortable but could not explain why, the feeling was just there.

In the margins of your journal, record what you think your intuition is telling you and then come back to those instances to see if what you felt or heard – your intuition – was right or whether it was something else, like impulse. In this way, you will begin to hone, develop, and trust your intuition.

Where Are You Returning From? Where Are You Going Next?
When we go on a journey of journaling, go on a retreat, spend an extended amount of time helping to care for someone, experience travel, or have been working on a project for a long time, we might come back or re-emerge feeling different than before embarking on the journey.

The challenge is that we may feel that no one understands us and what we have gone through. And, we might not fully understand what we are feeling or have gone through ourselves. We might sense or know that we need to make changes but may either not know which change to start with, feel overwhelmed with making any sort of change, or lack the support of family members, friends, colleagues, or others to implement and carry out the needed change. If that is the case, here are some ways I recommend to transition from where you are returning from, or have been, to how to find ways to proceed in your life going forward:

- Acknowledge how you feel and why and write about it in your journal
- Write ideas and plans for the future and action steps to take to see your plans take shape and become reality, even if the action or progress seem barely noticeable, small, overwhelming, or blocked
- Be strong in your faith that God will guide and protect you and provide the resources, people, timing, and support to you at the right moments along the way
- Have hope for the future each minute, hour, and day

A **Life Journal** can be a wonderful way to capture the beauty, hopes, plans, fears, and stories of your life and of others. Enjoy your journaling time with writing about these:

- Personal and Family Relationships
- Personal Journey
- Family History
- Decisions and Fear
- Acting with Courage
- Dreams, Hopes, Plans
- Intuition
- Where Are You Returning From? Where Are You Going Next?

21

Money/Finance Journal

"You must gain control over your money or the lack of it will forever control you."
– Dave Ramsey

In addition to having a budget, keeping a **Money/Finance Journal** can be an excellent way to jot down things you learn about money. You can write down your thoughts on money after reviewing resources such as articles, books, magazines, and podcasts.

Finding and Accessing Financial Resources
Maybe a friend or family member recommended a podcast, book, article, or course that is on personal finances. Make note of the name of the podcast, book, article, or course; listen to an episode; read a chapter or paragraph; or attend a class, and write down all of the things that stand out to you:

- Financial decisions or actions you need to make or take
- Research you want to do into an area within finances: budgeting, financial planning, wills, investing, real estate, etc.

- Other resources that were mentioned that you want to listen to, read, or watch
- Any questions you have for or information you need to get from financial professionals such as accountants, financial planners, lawyers, investment advisors, or others

Personal Versus Business Finances
Do you find that you approach personal and business finances in different ways? For example, are you more or less risk-averse when deciding on the use and investment of personal or business finances? If you find that there is a significant difference in one compared to the other, it could be that – in the case of owning or being part of a business – you have more advisors providing advice or maybe, in personal finances, there are more available funds to invest. Being aware of any differences you notice and writing about them can help you identify the areas where you need to improve or change how you handle personal or business finances.

Money Associations
You can take note of your thoughts and associations around money, both from what you learned and absorbed during childhood and how, as an adult, that has shaped how you manage your financial resources now. How you look after your financial resources includes all of these areas:

- Budgeting
- Saving
- Spending
- Giving
- Debt
- Investments

Some other areas in your money and finances to pause and consider include:

- If and when you have the impulse to shop (does this happen when you are feeling discouraged/disappointed/sad/lonely or when you want to celebrate or after you received a promotion?)
- How you feel when you spend versus save
- Any other feelings, emotions, behaviors, or patterns you are aware you have or notice with regards to money and financial topics

Money is a neutral entity – it is the attitude toward it that governs how it is handled. The Bible provides many insights on the relationship to money and instructions on matters related to finances. Here are just a few of the verses you will find there:

- "A good man leaveth an inheritance to his children's children: and the wealth of the sinner is laid up for the just." Proverbs 13:22 (KJV)
- "The greedy bring ruin to their households, but the one who hates bribes will live." Proverbs 15:27 (NIV)
- "The rich rule over the poor, and the borrower is slave to the lender." Proverbs 22:7 (NIV)
- "For the love of money is a root of all kinds of evil. Some people, eager for money, have wandered from the faith and pierced themselves with many griefs." 1 Timothy 6:10 (NIV)
- "Anyone who does not provide for their relatives, and especially for their own household, has denied the faith and is worse than an unbeliever." 1 Timothy 5:8 (NIV)

Approach to Budgeting
What is your approach to budgeting? Do you have a budget? If you have a partner or spouse, do both of you agree that a budget is an essential tool to handle finances? How do you and your partner approach budgeting as a couple – do both partners agree on decisions, does one spouse – perhaps the husband - give a monthly amount to pay all household expenses, does each family member receive a monthly amount just for their use, at their complete discretion? Did your parents have a budget when you were growing up and did you see how they discussed finances and made financial decisions? It is important to reflect on these questions, or others that come up in your journal to understand what influences shaped you over the years that affect how and why you budget.

Teaching Finances to Your Children
If you have children, it is essential to consider what money and financial examples and lessons you are showing and teaching to them. Take to your journal to write down what patterns you observe in your own finances that you want to pass on to your kids as well as those areas where you and your children can improve. You can also use your journal to list ideas for ways to teach your kids about money and write down their money- and finance-related questions to then find answers to.

Investments and More
Investing and saving for the future is part of good financial planning and stewardship. You might like to begin learning more about this area by watching videos, borrowing books from the library and buying books from bookstores, or taking classes or courses to become familiar with and gain confidence in investing. Journal about insights that you learn along the way.

Starting and regularly keeping a **Money/Finance Journal** will help you be wise with where you direct your financial resources. In this chapter, here are some ideas that were given for topics and areas to journal about:

- Finding and Accessing Financial Resources
- Personal Versus Business Finances
- Money Associations
- Approach to Budgeting
- Teaching Finances to Your Children
- Investments and More

22

Nature Journal

"Some old-fashioned things like fresh air and sunshine are hard to beat."
– Laura Ingalls Wilder

If you enjoy spending time outside or would like to learn more about what you see in nature, start a **Nature Journal** and take it along with you when you explore outdoors. Over time, you can look back at your journal and notice all that you have discovered and observed over weeks, months, or years.

A Variety of Forms and Interactions
Take your journal, perhaps an unlined one, or a sketchpad with you when you go on a walk around your neighborhood or for a nature walk. Record what you see, observe, and hear with these suggested materials:

- Colored pencils
- Pencils
- Pen and ink

- Crayons
- Highlighters

Capture your impressions, what you see and hear, and respond in many different forms such as:

- Poems
- Drawings
- Stories
- Letters
- Quotes

Ideas for ways to enjoy nature:

- Take an umbrella and go for a walk in the rain (be prepared, though, by wearing a raincoat and rubber boots)
- Notice the sound of footsteps in the snow – is it a crunch or a soft thud?
- What birds do you see in your area? Take a book or guide along to help you identify the birds that you see.

Sounds
Take your journal and go to a nearby park. Try writing while sitting next to water such as a lake, stream, creek, or fountain. Notice how sounds, such as the soft babbling stream of a creek, the powerful sound of a waterfall, the chirping of birds, or distant voices and footsteps affect how you feel and the way or what you write. Also, take note whether you prefer writing in nature earlier in the day – before the hustle and bustle starts – or during midday or later in the day – as to-dos and activities wind down.

Each time you go out into nature, try to notice a different sound. One time you might notice the melody of birds singing, another time it may be the bubbling of a creek, then the rustling of leaves, and after that the sound of the wind. There are many unique sounds to listen for each time you visit the vast playground known as nature.

Views and Observations
You may enjoy journaling while sitting on a bench that holds a view over a valley or ravine or maybe hills or mountains in the distance. You can include in your **Nature Journal** the colors of sunrises and sunsets, the texture of leaves and barks, and the variety of colorful flowers as part of your observation and description of nature and the outdoors.

You can take your journal with you whenever you go out into nature. Whether you go on a hike, go camping, or take a stroll through a park or in a neighborhood, there are always things you can find to observe. Things you might observe in nature are:

- New trees that have been planted
- A new path going through the park or one that you had not noticed before
- Ducks sitting by or swimming in the pond
- A butterfly sitting on top of a flower
- A ladybug on a blade of grass
- Clouds in the sky
- Scents such as fresh mountain air, the air from the ocean, or different scents in each of the seasons

Nature has been created beautifully by the Lord. Our **Nature Journals** can be a place where we record our praise and thanks to Him for His creation and marvelous works.

Writing and Images
Writing poems and short stories about nature are items to include in the pages of your nature notebook. Or perhaps you might prefer to copy your favorite poems or quotes about nature. Other ideas for things to include in your **Nature Journal** are:

- Photos of nature, both parks and outdoor spaces you have been to and those you wish to visit in the future
- Gardens and trails you want to travel to, both locally and farther away

A **Nature Journal** is your chance to spend time outside and observe and record what you notice. You can use your **Nature Journal** to record:

- A Variety of Forms and Interactions
- Sounds
- Views and Observations
- Writing and Images

23

Prayer/Faith/Bible Journal

"Faith gives you an inner strength and a sense of balance and perspective in life."
– Gregory Peck

"Whatever is true, whatever is noble, whatever is right, whatever is pure, whatever is lovely, whatever is admirable—if anything is excellent or praiseworthy—think about such things."
– Philippians 4:8 (NIV)

Before your time of journaling and thinking, ask the Lord to help you grow in knowledge and wisdom. God wants for you to share your thoughts with Him. He wants you to share and pour out your struggles and challenges. He wants you to praise Him during good times as well as tough times or rough patches. In this chapter, you will learn about ways to use a **Prayer/Faith/Bible Journal** to keep you encouraged on your faith journey.

Faith and Prayer
Both faith and prayer are part of an active spiritual life. In your journal, write down the dates of your prayer requests and others'

prayer requests, when and how prayers were answered, times when faith was exercised, and examples of the faith of others. You might be surprised or perhaps, at first, even disappointed in how a particular prayer was answered as it might not be the answer you were hoping for. However, there will also be plenty of times and instances when you will see a constant faithfulness in provision, and your trust and faith will grow.

You can also write down times and instances when you feel or notice that the timing of an event – such as running into a friend you have not seen in a while or a job lead from an unexpected person or source – is Providential and a blessing. In the same way, the striking colors of a sunrise or sunset can bring you to give thanks for the beauty of nature created by the One Who made it for our enjoyment.

Keeping a prayer journal or journal of your Christian faith walk can be a place to turn to when you want to be reminded of and encouraged that God is working in your life, and in others' lives, even when you do not see it. Your journal could also be a way for you to encourage others – by looking back on answered prayers, seeing how the Lord has provided for your needs, and how the timing of an event was right. You can then share how God has worked in your life and thus strengthen your faith and the faith of others.

Bible Reading and Bible Study
The Bible contains everything we need to know God, learn about Jesus, and help us live our lives on Earth. Keep your journal next to you as you read the Bible to write down:

- Verses to learn the meaning of or to memorize
- Stories that teach a lesson

- Promises to encourage or strengthen you and give you hope for the future
- Words to look up the definitions of
- Names and their meanings
- Events that took place and where and when
- Places that you want to understand the geography or setting of
- Prophecies that were told – who told them and when they were fulfilled
- Commands given and kept
- Anything else that stands out to you

You might like to research topics or areas of interest – for example, money matters, relationships, character traits, guarding your heart, etc. – to know what the Bible says about them and elaborate on those in your journal. Include insights from Bible commentaries, theology books, and other resources you find along with any new perspectives or interpretations you want to look into to understand more.

Your Life's Purpose
Some of the primary purposes of a Christian's life are to be reconciled to Jesus, to minister to other Christians, to share the Gospel with others, to fear and love God, and to keep His commands. Use your journal as a place to check in on this area of your life and write down prayers and Bible verses, ideas, and prompts that come to you to meditate and act on.

Favorite Hymns, Old and New
Hymns are a wonderful way to be reminded of Biblical truths and be encouraged when going through difficult or sad times in life. Write down favorite and memorable verses and choruses from your favorite hymns and Christian songs. You could look up and read the

biographies of the writers and composers of the hymns and songs you like to learn how God worked in their lives. Another idea is to use your journal to write and compose your own hymns.

Sermon Notes
Take a journal or notebook with you to church and note mentions of verses, books, and related chapters and stories shared during the sermon. After the sermon, you can look up these items to learn more and grow in your faith and understanding of the Bible and how it applies to your life.

Learning About Missionaries
Take the time to read and learn about the biographies and lives of missionaries across the centuries and in different countries. Use your journal as a place to respond to thoughts, feelings, and prayers that come up in relation to what you read and learn. In what ways have missionaries stayed strong in their faith while sharing their faith with others? How did God provide for them during trials and how did other believers meet the needs of missionaries? Do you know of any contemporary missionaries? How could you be an encouragement and support to them? What challenges have missionaries faced and overcome in the past and what challenges do they face these days?

Grow in your faith by keeping a **Prayer/Faith/Bible Journal** to record:

- Faith and Prayer
- Bible Reading and Bible Study
- Favorite Hymns, Old and New
- Sermon Notes
- Learning About Missionaries

24

Travel Journal

"Journal writing is a voyage to the interior."
– Christina Baldwin, *Life's Companion*

There is so much to look forward to and enjoy about traveling. You do not always have to fly to a destination or go somewhere abroad to travel. Indeed, there are many places to visit close to where we call home, whether in or just outside one's city, in one's state or province, and also in one's country.

Planning Future Trips and Setting Travel Goals
What are your plans and desires for travel? Perhaps you want to do a road trip through your state/province and visit all of the state/provincial or national parks. Or maybe you would prefer to do a bicycle tour through Europe.

This is where the fun of having a **Travel Journal** comes in. Make note of places you want to visit and your travel experiences. You can begin the process of planning your trip in a journal by jotting down the names of attractions or inns you want to visit or stay at as you come across them when reading newspapers, magazines, or online articles.

As you set travel goals, write down the things you need to do to prepare for any trip you are planning to make such as:

- What to pack
- Passports, documents, or other papers to have ready
- Maps and tourist guides of the towns/cities/regions you would like to visit
- Currency to have on hand
- Vaccinations
- Attractions to visit
- A list of accommodations and dates to stay there
- Anything else that would be helpful to ensure you are set to go

You can also write down the amount you need to save for your travel goals. Then, write down ideas for how to save that amount and record progress so that you can see that you are getting closer to achieving your goals.

Upon returning from traveling, take the time to review how the trip went – what worked and went well and what did not, what you enjoyed seeing that was or was not on your list, travel tips you learned, things to pack or leave at home next time, and whatever else comes to mind. Reviewing your trip in your journal and the information you take away after each trip can be beneficial when applied to planning future travels.

Travel Wisdom
What wisdom and advice have you received from other travelers about tips relating to packing and destinations or places you want to visit?

Or have you been given suggestions for transportation and lodging or accommodations? Write down those that you find are most interesting, relevant, or applicable to your travel goals and plans. Some tips or mentions will be a better fit depending on which part of the world you are preparing to travel to.

Taking Your Journal with You on Your Travels
Do you have a trip booked? Great! This is the perfect time to take your journal along for the ride, flight, hike, etc. (pun intended).

You will entertain many thoughts and encounter many objects, experiences, places, and more when traveling or on vacation. Set aside a few minutes in the morning, evening, or throughout the day to write down all that happens and what you feel. For example, what was it like touring the home of your favorite author? Did you feel relaxed as you enjoyed a morning latte on a sunny sidewalk café? Do you have new projects, plans, and ideas for things to do or change in your life or work on upon returning home? Going away for a short time is a fabulous opportunity for slowing down, reflecting, and hitting the reset button.

You can take the same journal along for all your travels or you could use a new journal for each of your trips. A pocket-size notebook may be more convenient as you travel. Whether on a backpacking trek, cross-country bicycling tour, six-month road trip, or another type of adventure, remember to bring your journal on the journey. It can be a pretty sweet way to relive moments from past travels, months or years down the road.

One day, you might decide to turn the reflections of your travel journal into a travel book. The description of sights, sounds, tastes, people, and activities will make your memories of travel that much more vivid and colorful.

Far Away Near
As much as it can be new and exciting to travel to other countries and continents, remember that there is so much to discover and explore within driving distance of where you call home. Places and things to see close by might include:

- Staying overnight at a hotel or campground you have never stayed at before but always wanted to try
- Visiting a newly opened business or store or attending their grand opening
- Taking a road trip or driving down a highway you have never driven on before but want to explore
- Going to a gallery or museum to see an exhibit
- Going on a farm tour and learning about the farms in your county or state or province and what grows in your area
- Exploring a new-to-you park path or park you have always wanted to walk, or changing things up and trying a different route on your next bicycle trip or walk
- Visiting a landmark or a historical park or village to learn more about the history in your area
- Attending a festival or concert

There are many ways to travel, learn, and explore in your local area. As you discover places, things, and events nearer to home, make sure to keep your eyes open to truly observe and notice what is around you. What does it feel like to be a tourist in your area? What have you learned about your area that you did not know before? Do you feel more connected to your geographical area by learning more about the history or tourist attractions that are nearby?

It is often a surprise to those who have lived in the same place for 10, 15, or 20 years that it has either taken them that long to visit local parks or museums, etc. or that they were not even aware that a place existed until they took a different turnoff one day and saw a sign by the road.

Time Travel
An aspect of a **Travel Journal** that you might not have considered is that it provides the means for time travel, in years to come, by going back in time. By capturing sights, sounds, experiences, interactions and meetings, and snippets of talk along your travels, you will be able to go back and relive and re-experience the highlights and locations you saw and the people you met along the way.

Think about it – in the future, to go back in time. How neat is that? You will be able to recall laughs, smiles, tears, hugs, kisses. You will remember the times you felt afraid or scared or when you felt very adventurous and brave. Should life circumstances change in the future, due to stage of life, financial situation, etc., you can still enjoy memories through your travel journals. Many years later, on a sunny afternoon or rainy day, you can take out your travel journals and have all of this to travel back in time to and perhaps share your travel memories with children, grandchildren, and other relatives.

Areas and topics to explore in a **Travel Journal** can be:

- Planning Future Trips and Travel Goals
- Travel Wisdom
- Taking Your Journal with You On Your Travels
- Far Away Near
- Time Travel

III

Part 3: Hands-on Workbook - How to Sustain Your Journaling Practice

Part 3 presents a workbook with questions to ask and space to answer. The questions are grouped into categories: The Place and Space Where You Journal, Goals and Reasons for Journaling, Time to Journal, Socialization and Support Systems, and Health and Wellness. By writing down answers to these questions, you will develop a better understanding of your journaling preferences and goals, changes to make as you begin to journal, and potential challenges to sustaining a journaling practice.

25

The Place and Space Where You Journal

1) Is there a place that you find the most conducive to journaling, such as a sunlit window seat, an outdoor porch or patio, in a favorite armchair, a basement office, or elsewhere?
If you do not currently have a place or space where you can journal, take the time to think about the possible areas where you could do so. Write down any ideas that come to mind for possible places and spaces to go to, be in, or use when you want to journal:

* * *

2) What do you need or appreciate in the space where you journal? Circle those that you appreciate and/or need:

a) Natural and/or direct light

b) A view of hills, water, or mountains
c) Warmth and heat
d) Peace and quiet
e) Plenty of space
f) A comfortable chair
g) A big desk
h) Cozy nook
i) Other (e.g., a bookshelf, counter space, writing/art supplies, artwork, inspirational quotes):

If you do not have some of the above in your journaling space, are there ways you can enjoy them, even if on a limited basis? For example, if you like to have a view of hills, mountains, or water while journaling but your space does not have that, then can you find a park with a pond or a hill overlooking a lake or with a view of mountains in the distance? Or can you add photos of hills, mountains, and water to your journaling space? Write down your solutions below:

* * *

3) What are ways in which you can personalize your journaling space? Write down your ideas here (look at your ideas in point 2 above):

1.

2.

3.

* * *

4) In addition to your journal, are there any other items that you need close by? Circle the items below:

a) Diffuser
b) Candles
c) A lamp
d) Blanket
e) Water or tea
f) Books on journaling
g) Flowers
h) Photos
i) A mat or mattress
j) Other:

* * *

5) Are there any changes or improvements you need to make to your journaling space at home? If yes, write them down in the space below:

a. Change to be made:

Complete by:

b. Change to be made:

Complete by:

c. Change to be made:

Complete by:

26

Goals and Reasons for Journaling

1) Why do you want to journal? Circle those that are important to you:

a) To express and show your gratitude
b) To capture all the joy in your life
c) To record happenings and events in your life
d) To help you make decisions
e) To explore the options, possibilities, and paths you could choose to take, pursue, or follow
f) Other:

* * *

2) What are your goals, both short-term and long-term, for journaling?

Short-term goals for journaling…

Long-term goals for journaling...

* * *

3) Brainstorm ways to stay on track with and reach your journaling goals (for example, get organized, set a time to journal, etc.):

Do you need to make any changes to reach your journaling goals?

GOALS AND REASONS FOR JOURNALING

***

4) How often do you currently write down your goals? How often do you examine your goals to make sure that you are on track to reach them, both in journaling and other areas of life?

***

5) Of the ways to journal about goals shared in the **Goals Journal** chapter, which ones did you find most helpful and which ones would be most helpful for you to implement?

- Timeline of Goals
- Time
- Energy
- Learning and Growing
- Supporting Others
- Supporting Yourself
- Vision Board

27

Time to Journal

1) At what part(s) of the day do you find it best to journal? Circle the time(s) of the day when you journal best:

a) Early morning: 5 a.m. – 8 a.m.
b) Morning: 8 a.m. – 12 p.m.
c) Early afternoon: 12 p.m. – 2 p.m.
d) Afternoon: 2 p.m. – 5 p.m.
e) Evening: 5 p.m. – 8 p.m.
f) Late evening: 8 p.m. – 12 a.m.
g) Wee morning: 12 a.m. – 5 a.m.

* * *

2) How much time each day or week or on the weekend can you set aside to journal? Circle the amount of time(s) you have each day or week:

a) 5-10 minutes each day/week
b) 15 minutes each day/week

c) 30 minutes each day/week
d) 45 minutes each day/week
e) 60 minutes each day/week
f) 60 minutes on the weekend
g) 120 minutes on the weekend

* * *

3) If you need to set aside more time in your schedule to allow for regular and dedicated journaling time, how will you rearrange or what changes will you make to your schedule? Will you say no to one or two commitments and if so, which one(s)? What are you willing to give up?

* * *

4) Do you need to schedule your journaling times on a calendar so that they are visible and blocked off from other requests that may come up? Do you need to use a clock or watch to ensure you journal for the amount of time you have set aside for it? Write down below whether you need to acquire a calendar, clock, etc. that will allow you to see your journaling times and how much journaling time you have left:

* * *

5) Describe – in as much detail as possible – your ideal journaling time. Here are some questions to get you started: How much time do you have set aside for journaling each day? Do you have music playing or a water fountain on in the background? What do you do before and after journaling?

28

Socialization and Support Systems

1) Is there a writing or journaling group you might like to join where you can find support and encouragement on the journaling journey? Check with local writing groups and look online to find available options. Write down the possibilities below:

* * *

2) Are there classes or workshops on journaling that you would like to attend to learn more about journaling? Reach out to writing groups in your area and search online to learn about classes and workshops

offered. Jot down the things you would like to learn more about on journaling:

* * *

3) Look at the books on journaling and personal journals written by others (see the **Resources** section) and write down which one(s) you would like to read.
Reading these can provide support, encouragement, and inspiration.

* * *

SOCIALIZATION AND SUPPORT SYSTEMS

4) What are some ways that family and friends can help out at home or elsewhere, so that you would have the support needed to journal regularly? Write them below and share them with family and friends:

* * *

5) Who is your cheering team (i.e., those who support, encourage, listen, and provide feedback) from among your family and friends? Write the names of five people who are your cheering group and what you appreciate about them:

1. Name:

I appreciate that:

2. Name:

I appreciate that:

3. Name:

I appreciate that:

4. Name:

I appreciate that:

5. Name:

I appreciate that:

29

Health and Wellness

1) What are the ways you would like your journaling practice to support or add to your health and wellness journey? Circle the reasons in the list below and/or write your own reasons:

a) Add joy to your life
b) Release stress
c) Get to know yourself
d) Find purpose in life
e) Become aware of patterns and habits of behavior and thought
f) Have accountability in changing unsupportive behaviors and thoughts
g) Identify/learn about the stressors in your life and how to minimize or remove them
h) Support your overall mental, emotional, physical, and spiritual health
i) Other:

* * *

2) What are your goals, both short-term and long-term, for spiritual growth, health and wellness, etc.?

Short-term goals for spiritual growth, health and wellness, etc....

Long-term goals for spiritual growth, health and wellness, etc....

* * *

3) In addition to supporting your health and wellness through journaling, what other habits or rituals can you begin or continue along your health and wellness journey? Circle from the list below and/or write your own reasons:

a) Start your day with a glass of warm lemon water
b) Drink a glass of greens
c) Finish your day with a cup of tea
d) Read a relaxing, encouraging book
e) Go for a walk
f) Jump on a rebounder trampoline once or twice a day
g) Other:

* * *

4) Can journaling on a regular basis help you in any of these ways?

a) Decrease stress
b) Decrease boredom
c) Decrease loneliness
d) Reduce bad habits
e) Increase creativity
f) Find purpose
g) Increase productivity
h) Other:

* * *

5) How will you know that you are making progress in achieving your health and wellness goals?

IV

Resources

30

Books

Books - on Journaling

Creative Journal Writing: The Art and Heart of Reflection by Stephanie Dowrick
Journal to the Self: Twenty-Two Paths to Personal Growth by Kathleen Adams, M.A.
Life's Companion: Journal Writing as a Spiritual Practice by Christina Baldwin
Writer with a Day Job by Aine Greaney (specifically, Chapter 5: Journal Writing)
100% Happiness: A Guided Journal to Enhance Your Daily Life by Raphaelle Giordano
Dot Journaling – A Practical Guide: How to Start and Keep the Planner, To-Do List, and Diary That'll Actually Help You Get Your Life Together by Rachel Wilkerson Miller
The Bullet Journal Method: Track the Past, Order the Present, Design the Future by Ryder Carroll
Journaling For Joy: Writing Your Way to Personal Growth and Freedom by Joyce Chapman

The Great Book of Journaling: How Journal Writing Can Support a Life of Wellness, Creativity, Meaning and Purpose by Eric Maisel and Lynda Monk

Books - Journal Memoirs (Journals Written by Others)

The Journal Keeper: A Memoir by Phyllis Theroux
Roughing It in the Bush by Susanna Moodie
Her Life, Letters, and Journals by Louisa May Alcott
Journals by Winston Churchill, Henry David Thoreau, and others

Books - on Creativity, Inspiration, and Ideas

Write for Life: Creative Tools for Every Writer by Julia Cameron
The Artist's Way: A Spiritual Path to Higher Creativity by Julia Cameron
The Creative Life: True Tales of Inspiration by Julia Cameron
Fearless Creating: A Step-by-Step Guide to Starting and Completing Your Work of Art by Eric Maisel
Keep Going: 10 Ways to Stay Creative in Good Times and Bad by Austin Kleon
100 Side Hustles: Unexpected Ideas for Making Extra Money Without Quitting Your Day Job by Chris Guillebeau
Creative, Inc.: The Ultimate Guide to Running a Successful Freelance Business by Meg Mateo Ilasco and Joy Deangdeelert Cho

Books - on Work

- Working from Home

Home at the Office: Working Remotely as a Way of Life by Barbori Garnet
Great Pajama Jobs: Your Complete Guide to Working from Home by Kerry

Hannon

The Ultimate Guide to Remote Work: How to Grow, Manage, and Work with Remote Teams by Wade Foster and the Zapier Team

Work Together Anywhere: A Handbook on Working Successfully for Individuals, Teams & Managers by Lisette Sutherland & K. Janene-Nelson

Will Work from Home: Earn the Cash – Without the Commute by Tory Johnson and Robyn Freedman Spizman

- Entrepreneurial Ideas

100 Side Hustles: Unexpected Ideas for Making Extra Money Without Quitting Your Day Job by Chris Guillebeau

Creative, Inc.: The Ultimate Guide to Running a Successful Freelance Business by Meg Mateo Ilasco and Joy Deangdeelert Cho

- Retirement/Second Career

How to Retire Happy, Wild, and Free: Retirement Wisdom That You Won't Get From Your Financial Advisor by Ernie J. Zelinski

The Joy of Not Working: A Book for the Retired, Unemployed, and Overworked by Ernie J. Zelinski

Start Your Own Home Business After 50: How to Survive, Thrive, and Earn the Income You Deserve! by Robert W. Bly

31

Websites

- Center for Journal Therapy: www.JournalTherapy.com
- International Association for Journal Writing: www.iajw.org
- Bullet Journal: www.BulletJournal.com

32

Dualities

As you journal, you may notice that many dualities, contrasts, or opposites appear in what and how you write. That is okay. Life is full of these instances so it makes sense that they would be captured in our journal writing.

While the below is not exhaustive, examples of dualities, contrasts, or opposites are:

1. Asking Questions – Finding/Discovering Answers
2. Joy – Sadness
3. Laughter – Tears
4. Hope – Despair
5. Memories of Childhood – Realities of Adulthood
6. Life – Death
7. Light – Dark
8. Health – Sickness
9. Beginning – Finishing
10. Start – End
11. Fast – Slow

12. Past – Future
13. New – Old
14. Moving Forward – Stuck/Stalled/Stopped
15. Younger – Older
16. Open – Closed
17. Fresh – Withered
18. Love – Hate
19. Warm/Hot – Cold
20. Energy – Lethargy
21. Open Vision – Narrow-sightedness
22. Free – Trapped/Confined
23. Positive – Negative
24. Strength – Weakness
25. Wet – Dry
26. Courage – Fear
27. Faith – Doubt
28. Large – Small
29. Exploring – Passing by
30. Welcoming – Ignoring
31. Caring – Neglecting
32. Truth – Lies
33. Right – Wrong
34. Rich – Poor
35. Social – Withdrawn
36. Logical – Emotional
37. Observing – Participating
38. Known – Unknown

33

Days and Holidays to Journal About

- Birthdays (yours and other family members')
- Weddings
- Anniversaries
- Graduations
- Reunions
- New Year's Eve/New Year's Day
- Valentine's Day
- Easter
- Mother's/Father's Day
- Siblings' Day
- Grandparents' Day
- Births
- Deaths
- Thanksgiving
- Christmas
- Canada Day/Independence Day/Your country's day
- Remembrance Day/Memorial Day/Veterans Day

34

Journal Prompts and Questions

- What thoughts begin to race in your mind as soon as you settle down to journal? Why?
- How is your journaling different or the same when you are on holiday compared to at home? What is the reason for any differences?
- What are some of your behaviors and patterns that you would like to change for the better, both for yourself and others (spouse, children, grandchildren, etc.)? What is a first step or two to take to make those changes?
- Growing up, what was your relationship like with your mother and/or your father? With other family members? Why were the relationships and interactions with your parents (and other family members) the way they were?
- Did any form of abuse – physical, emotional, financial, etc. – occur in family relationships? Have you been able to identify specific instances? Have you sought help to work through topics or issues in order to understand better what has happened?
- Who are you a product of? Who or what, including ideas, events,

traditions, standards, and expectations, have contributed to make you who you are today?
- Do you like who you are now? If not, why not? What do you need to change and how are you going to make that change?
- Write a separate list each for your favorite books, art, games, songs, movies, and TV shows. What do they have in common – author, character, actor, and/or theme or subject matter? Do certain feelings or themes run through the lists? Why or why not?
- What is your prayer for today? This week?
- What do you want to learn more about and study in the Bible? Which Bible verses do you want to memorize? How will memorizing Bible verses help you grow and be strong in your faith?
- What are ways you can stay strong and be encouraged in your faith and in pursuing and achieving your goals, even in the face of disappointment, discouragement, or loneliness?

35

A to Z of Journaling Prompts

Advice: Whose advice do you regret taking or wish you had not taken? Why? What was the outcome or result? Whose advice are you glad you took? Why? What was the outcome or result?

Business: Is there a business you have thought about starting? Would it be an online business or have a brick-and-mortar presence?

Choices: What choices and decisions do you need to make in the next week, month, and year? How does journaling help you make choices? Courage: Do you make decisions with courage? Are there times in your life you have shown courage or been courageous? Who do you admire for acting with courage?

Decisions: Do you find it easy or hard/difficult/challenging to make decisions? Are there certain areas of decision-making or topics/subjects – financial, travel, job, health – that you find easier or more straightforward to make than others?

Excellence: How do you show excellence in your work, at home, and to your family/friends/community/neighborhood? What does it mean to you to excel and do your best at work/in your career, in relationships, and other areas of your life?

Faith: What strengthens your faith and walk with God? Is it prayer, reading the Bible, memorizing scripture verses, singing hymns, and/or attending church? What are times in your life when having a strong faith has seen you through or helped you endure through challenging circumstances or events?

Fear: What is fear asking? What does fear want? What are the gifts that fear brings? Do you make decisions with some amount of fear, based on what-ifs or unknowns, or feel fear once you have made a decision? Where and how has fear influenced a decision in the past?

Focus: Do you notice that you come back to a certain topic or write a lot about a particular time in your life? It could be from your past – specific memories or experiences from your childhood. Or maybe it's a previous relationship that you seem to come back to in your journal. Take the time to know why and what steps you might need to take to work through and/or move on.

Freedom: What does freedom mean to you…
  - As a citizen?
  - In work (flexible hours, choice of location, own business, working on contract)?
  - To have choice in education, healthcare, and/or where you live?

Goals: What support – encouragement from others, time, financial resources, space – do you need from others and for you to be able to reach your goals? How can you show support to others to help them reach their goals?

Home: Which places throughout your life have truly felt like home?

Who or what contributed to making each place feel like home?

Ideas: Where/how/in what location(s) do you get ideas? What environments are most conducive for you to get your best ideas?

Journaling: Are there areas of your journaling that need changing, improving, or more creative expression such as using colored pens? What do you enjoy about the way you journal now and your current journaling routine?

Knowledge: What areas or subjects do you have lots of knowledge in? Which subjects or topics would you like to acquire more knowledge of and why?

Love: What does it mean to you to be in love? How is love shown or demonstrated in healthy relationships and friendships? How do you know that it is a healthy relationship when you are in love? When and how have you been disappointed in love? How does it make you feel?

Money: What is your relationship to and with money like? Describe how it makes you feel - nervous, excited, cautious, powerful – and why. Where do you go or turn to find wise guidance on money matters? What action(s) do you need to take in your finances – find and work with a financial advisor, make and stick to a budget, start or increase saving, and/or learning about investing?

Nature: Do you like nature? Why or why not? What aspects do you like – order and symmetry, fragrances, vistas – or do not like – stings, bites, changing temperatures?

Obey: Who or what are you willing/happy/reluctant to obey and why?

Principles: What are your principles and why? What do you stand for and why? What do you believe in and why?

Questions: What questions do you find yourself asking, both of yourself and others? Are there questions you seem to return to or repeat on a regular basis? When you need to find answers, which sources do you turn to?

Relationships: Which relationships – with your parents, siblings, extended family, friends, teachers, co-workers, managers – have had the biggest effect, either positive or negative, on your life? Why?

Shed Light On: These are all topics you could write about in your journal, whether something from the present or a time or happening or thoughts from the past, that you now find yourself ready to write about and shed light on:

- Health and healing
- First love
- Preparing for the future
- Loss of a loved one
- Anticipating the future
- First job
- Moving on
- Job loss
- Forgiveness
- Beloved or memorable pets
- College/post-secondary years
- What you wanted to be when you grew up
- Relationship with or influence of mother and father in or on your life

Silence: How often do you let yourself enjoy several minutes, or even an hour, of silence? Do you feel comfortable in quiet and calm surroundings or do you feel that something is missing? Why or why not?

Sweeping Under the Rug: What are you "sweeping under the rug" in your life? Those would be the things you are avoiding or ignoring in your life.

Travel: How do you feel when traveling – excited, nervous, and/or scared? Which situations produce these feelings?

Time: What is taking you more time to do, complete, research, etc., than it should? Why?

Undo: If you could undo and then redo something for the better, what would it be and why?

Vision: What is your vision for your life? Do you have a clearer vision of certain areas of your life over other areas? If so, which ones and why?

Weaknesses: What are your weaknesses – do you know what they are but have a hard time admitting to them? When or in what ways do your weaknesses surface or show up? Brainstorm ideas for how you can both acknowledge and overcome your weaknesses as well as learn from them, apologize when needed, and grow stronger and more self-confident.

Words: What words do you think about or associate with your journal or journaling and why? Some examples include:

- Loyal
- Nourishing

- Well-being
- A friend
- Ideas
- Trust
- Safe
- Supportive
- Challenging
- Overwhelming
- Solution-oriented
- Problem-solving
- Comforting
- Routine
- Mindfulness
- Creativity
- Health
- Truthfulness

X-ray: In what ways are you using journaling to "x-ray" - see through - a situation or issue?

Xylophone: Just as there are different notes and melodies in music, what are the different melodies in your life? What areas or times have been softer, louder, quicker, slower, harmonious, or melodious?

Years: Do you feel like some years of your life have gone by faster while others seem to have dragged on? Why or why not?

Zig Zags: Have there been any zig zags in your life that surprised you? Why? Were the zig zags, or detours, the result of decisions you have made or unforeseen happenings?

36

Journal to Rise (aka Start Your Day)

Upon waking, start the day with journaling and try including some of the suggested activities and rituals or routines below:

- <u>Monday:</u> Journaling followed by gentle stretches or light exercise such as rebounding and lifting dumbbells
- <u>Tuesday:</u> A time of reading and then journaling in response to what you read
- <u>Wednesday:</u> A morning teatime enjoyed in the early morning light while you journal
- <u>Thursday:</u> Making time for creative expression and journaling about it afterward
- <u>Friday:</u> Indoor or outdoor gardening, depending on the climate and the season, and journaling about observations and thoughts on what is growing
- <u>Saturday:</u> A morning bath time followed by journaling
- <u>Sunday:</u> Enjoy either a day of rest or a shorter time of journaling to reflect back on the week and to recharge and prepare for the week

37

Journal to Bed (aka Finish Your Day)

As you prepare for bed, include journaling as part of your time to let go of stress and relax before enjoying a restful, restorative sleep. Pair journaling with calming activities and rituals or routines, such as:

- Monday: Yin Yoga – holding restorative poses for a longer time in order to gently and slowly increase stretching and range of motion – accompanied by candlelight and/or soft music and journaling
- Tuesday: Tea – chamomile, lavender, peppermint – and journaling
- Wednesday: A warm, relaxing bath during the middle of the week followed by a time of journaling
- Thursday: A time of reading an inspiring, encouraging – faith-based, autobiography, heart-warming fiction – book and journaling
- Friday: Enjoy a massage – hot stone, aromatherapy, relaxation, etc. – and journal afterward
- Saturday: A relaxing creative pursuit such as drawing, painting, knitting, scrapbooking, baking, etc. and then taking time to journal
- Sunday: Either enjoy a day of rest or journal for a shorter length of time in order to focus on recharging and preparing for the week

38

Sample Journaling Retreat Day

Treat yourself to a retreat day that includes not only journaling but other self-care practices that are sure to both relax and refresh you while renewing your energy, confidence, and strength!

Wake up:
Glass of warm lemon water
Glass of green powder
Jump on a rebounder trampoline for 10 minutes

Throughout the day:
Journal – morning, afternoon, and evening pages
Yoga and/or stretches
Fresh juice
Meals and snacks consisting of fruit, nuts, seeds, fresh and lightly steamed veggies, large colorful salad
Herbal tea
Take a walk outside
Go for a massage
Read books that uplift, encourage, and motivate you

Run an air diffuser using essential oils

<u>Before bed:</u>
Herbal tea
Try self-massage
Enjoy a relaxing bath time
Apply essential oils for a restful and peaceful sleep

39

Article - Journaling for Writers

Journaling for Writers
By Barbori Garnet

Some Reasons Writers Should Journal
With already not enough time to get in all the writing needed to work on story outlines, meet book deadlines for editors, publishers, and others, why should writers add journaling to their writing schedule?

Journaling is a great place to get clarity
Because, a journal is a great place to work out feelings and emotions in life in such a way that it provides clarity to what a writer may then decide to include in a story. A journal can be the first place to go and seek solace in to sort through what you have experienced and felt before it goes anywhere else.

Another excellent reason for writers to journal is to write down your goals, plans, and dreams for you as a writer and for your writing. This can be especially encouraging when you feel stuck or are losing direction in your writing. You can go back to your journal and review your goals and plans. Then, you can journal more or make a new journal entry about whether and why your writing goals have changed and the steps to take to reach your goals.

Journaling may help you notice moments of inspiration

A third reason to journal is to record and remember moments in your day-to-day life. It may seem that not much happens in your life. However, by taking the time to write down daily occurrences, you can look back and notice happenings and events. You might notice things such as when you had the most inspiration and the circumstances causing this burst of creativity, what day you submitted your query or manuscript to an agent or publisher, or when you were accepted into a residency, anthology, or other publications or opportunities. These can be encouraging to you as writer. In addition, keeping a journal of your life's moments can be a help should you decide in the future to write a memoir or autobiography of your life or describe a certain event or time in your life.

Journaling can be rewarding

Journaling for writers can be very rewarding as well as relaxing. With so many good reasons and benefits for writers to journal – capturing feelings, goals, and daily happenings – this will soon become an enjoyable addition to your daily writing routine.

Originally published in Opal Writers Magazine's digital magazine on July 5, 2022. Reprinted with permission from Opal Publishing.

40

Article - Support Your Health with a Health Journal

Support Your Health with a Health Journal
By Barbori Garnet

Keeping a health journal gives you space and guidance wherein to write down things you notice about your health. By writing down things you observe about your health, it frees you from the stress of having to remember and recall things later on. Instead, you can refer back to your journal and know exactly the day, and maybe even the time of day, when you ate a particular food, did many repetitions of a certain exercise, or felt something specific in your body.

Things it might include:
Because a health journal should be a tool to support you in your health journey, make sure it is manageable and enjoyable rather than becoming one more thing adding the feeling of pressure to your to-do list. Your health journal is yours. Things to include might be:

- the foods you eat and how they make you feel or how they are

helping you achieve your health goals
- the quality and length of your sleep
- in what ways your emotional state affects your overall health
- external factors that might be affecting your health such as a busy schedule
- when and what kind of exercise you do and how that particular exercise affects how you feel

What format works for you?
Choose a format that works for you, whether print or digital. A smaller size of journal can fit into your pocket or bag while a digital version can be an app on your phone, both of which you can take with you wherever you go. By being able to take your health journal with you wherever you go, it makes it portable and accessible at any time. Keep your journal in the same place so that you know where it is and it is easy for you to find.

In your journal, make plans for ways to make progress towards reaching your health goals. Include action steps to take as well as those you have already tried. Record books, podcasts, and webinars you read and listen to on health topics and jot down important points. Write down questions that come up and things you want to look into and research further.

Review
Take the time to look over what you have written in your health journal. This is important so that you can determine what is working, notice any patterns of concern that need addressing, and change what is not working.

When is the best time to journal? Setting aside some minutes in the evening could be a good time to recollect things about your health that you remember from the day. During the summer months, that might mean enjoying the warmth and gentle glow of the setting sun while writing. Or choose the quiet time before everybody is up to record thoughts from the previous day.

Take the opportunity to write about your health in a journal. Give health journaling a try for a while to see if it is a fit for you and the ways in which it can assist you in supporting your health. Once you start journaling, you will discover the many benefits it offers to journal writers.

Originally published in Opal Rising Magazine's digital magazine on July 12, 2022. Reprinted with permission from Opal Publishing.

41

Book Club Discussion Guide

1. Which type of journal would you most like to try and why?
2. How much time do you think is the minimum needed for a regular – daily or weekly – journaling practice?
3. What is your ideal place or space to journal? Take the time to describe it. What do you like about it? Are there any changes that need to be made to make your current journaling space more ideal?
4. Do you find it easier to journal at a certain time of day, or during warmer or cooler weather or seasons?
5. What fears or obstacles might someone encounter prior to starting to journal or during regular journaling? How can the fears and obstacles be overcome?
6. Do you need to be part of a community that provides support to sustain a journaling practice?

42

A Little Help from Friends and Readers

I appreciate the support and help from friends, readers, and fans alike!

If you enjoyed this book, please leave a review on Amazon.com, Amazon.ca, and Goodreads.com by going to the book's page or visit my author page. Even a short review, of one or two sentences, would be a great help. Reviews help others find out about and learn more about my book.

To follow along on my writing journey, I hope you will visit my website www.BarboriGarnet.com and join by subscribing to my e-newsletter.

Thank you!
    Barbori Garnet

V

Index

Index

A

Adventures, 54
Answers, 10-11, 37-38
Art, Artwork, 26-28, 75-84, 117-118
Articles, 41-42

B

Behaviors, 95, 123-124, 131
Bible, 138-141
Books, 15, 41-42, 44-45, 117-119, 169-171
Budgeting, 132
Business, 61-74, 130

C

Candles, 26
Career, 61-74, 82, 115-116
Classes, 42, 80-82, 83, 88-90
Challenges, 53, 72
Changes, 51-52, 72

Character, 45, 118-119
Children, 22, 90-92, 132
Choices, 14, 66
Coach, Business or Career, 63
Communication, 28-29, 47-48, 107
Community, 40, 40-42
Courage, 50, 126
Courses, 42, 88-90
Creativity, 75-84

D

Decisions, 33, 45-47, 51-52, 126
Detours, 16
Diaries, 94-95
Diet, 110-111
Diffuser, Air, 25-26
Disappointment, 10, 36, 86, 124-125
Drawing, 26-28, 63-64, 76, 78-80, 134-135
Dreams, 85-87, 127

E

Education, 88-93
Emotions, 10, 28-29, 31-39, 52-53, 67, 131, 173-174
Energy, 33-34, 102-103
Essential Oils, 25-26, 34
Exercise, 33, 44, 111

F

Faith, 131, 139-142
Family, 22, 66, 92, 94-96, 123-124, 125-26, 132, 161
Fear, 32-33, 126

Feelings, 10, 33-34, 37, 51, 131
Finances, 64-65, 129-133
Fitness, 111, 164
Food, 110-111
Fragrances, 25-26, 98-99
Friend, Friends, Friendship, 11-12, 49-50, 52-53, 159-162
Future, 127, 128, 142-143
Future Log, 15

G

Gardening, 97-100
Goals, 87, 101-105, 142-143, 153-155
Gratitude, 106-109
Growing, Growth, 13, 103-104

H

Handwriting, 21, 27
Health, 17, 110-116, 163-165
Health Concerns/Issues, 35
Health Transition or Impact, 69-70, 115-116
History, Family, 94-96, 125-126
Holidays, 34, 175
Home Maintenance, 99-100
Homeschooling, 90-92
Hope, 127, 128
Hymns, 140-141

I

Ideas, 64-65, 117-118
Images, 137
Insight, 10-11

Interests, 117-122
Interviews, 34, 62
Intuition, 127
Investments, 132

J

Job Interviews, 34, 62
Journaling, Bullet, 15
Journey, 12-13, 30, 124-125
Joys, 28, 52-53, 125

K

L

Language, 120
Laughter, 52-53
Learning, 88-93, 103-104, 120
Letters, 27, 94-95, 135
Life, 55-56, 88-90, 123-128, 140
Light, 6, 25, 149
Lists, 27, 49
Live, 13

M

Memoirs, 41, 170
Men, Journaling for, 43-50
Money, 129-133, 143
Movies, 118-119
Music, 21, 117-118

N

Nature, 4-5, 134-137

O

Obstacles, 31-39
Organization, Organized, 14-15
Overwhelm, 35-36

P

Patterns, Family, 95
Personalize your Journal, 26-28
Pets, 21-22
Places to Journal, 4-5, 8, 32, 149-152
Plans, 127, 128, 142-143
Portable, 9-10
Practical, 9-10
Prayer, 138-141
Priorities, 15-16
Prompts, 176-183

Q

Questions, 13-14, 113-115
Quiet, 22

R

Reading, 41-42, 44-45, 117-118, 169-171
Reasons to Journal, 17-19, 153-155
Recipes, 110-111
Reflection, 17, 143
Relationships, 48-49, 123-124
Resources, 129-130, 169-194

Responsibilities, 44-45
Retirement, 70-71, 120-121
Retreat, 186-187
Returning, 127-128
Risk, 38
Roles, 44-45,
Routine, 20-23, 184-185

S

Seasons, 54-56, 102
Self-confidence, 12
Senses, 29-30
Sermon, 141
Sounds, 22, 135-136
Strength, 50
Stress, 70, 82-83, 115
Support, 40-42, 50, 104-105, 159-162

T

Tea, 6, 20
Technology, 65-66
Time, Times, 17, 72, 80-82, 102, 146, 156-158
Timeline, 101-102
Tone, 28-29
Traditions, 95-96
Travel, 142-146
Trips, 142-143

U

INDEX

V
Views, 136
Vision Board, 105, 155
Voice, 28-29

W
Water, 5, 22
Websites, 172
Wellness, 17, 163-165
Wisdom, 10-11, 143-144
Work, 43-46, 61-74
Workbook, 149-165
Work Environment, 67-68
Work From Home, 62-63
Writing, 22, 107, 137

X

Y
Year, 54-55, 101

Z

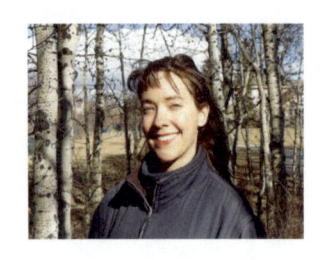

About the Author

Barbori Garnet has been journaling for many years. She has enjoyed the personal insights and wellness benefits derived from journaling.

Barbori is the author of *Home at the Office: Working Remotely as a Way of Life* (Atmosphere Press, 2021). She is a writer, artist, musician, and gardener based in Alberta.

Her other interests include reading, tennis, and enjoying cups of tea with family and friends.

To book a journaling consultation or workshop and to learn about journaling resources and support, visit Barbori online at www.BarboriGarnet.com.

You can connect with me on:
- https://barborigarnet.com
- https://www.facebook.com/barborigarnet
- https://www.instagram.com/barborigarnet

Also by Barbori Garnet

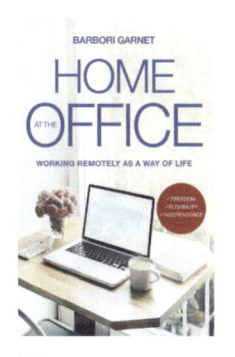

Home at the Office: Working Remotely as a Way of Life

What if I told you that working remotely can lead to increased freedom, flexibility, and independence in your life?

Home at the Office: Working Remotely as a Way of Life will help you:

Work remotely through any age and stage of life

Understand the work-from-home mindset

Learn the skills and character traits needed for remote work

Discover the 7 different types of working from home

Gain insights and secrets into how 10 extraordinary workers from home across North America succeed and face challenges in their remote work

Bringing over 10 years of work-from-home experience in writing, marketing, and music, Barbori Garnet invites you to join her as she shares how you can enjoy the rewards of freedom, flexibility, and independence found by working remotely.

Manufactured by Amazon.ca
Bolton, ON